PCOS Diet and Cookbook Recipe for Women:

The Ultimate 100+ Delicious and PCOS-friendly recipes

Dr. Mary K. Clubb

Table Of Content

Contents

1.0 Introduction to PCOS and Nutrition

Polycystic ovarian syndrome (PCOS) is a hormonal condition that affects women of reproductive age. Women with PCOS may face several symptoms, including irregular periods, increased facial and body hair, acne, weight gain, and trouble becoming pregnant. PCOS is also related to a higher chance of acquiring health disorders such as type 2 diabetes, heart disease, and endometrial cancer.

Although there is no treatment for PCOS, there are lifestyle adjustments that may help manage symptoms and minimize the risk of related health concerns. One of the essential lifestyle modifications for people with PCOS is food.

The introduction offers a summary of the major nutrients that are vital for women with PCOS, such as:

Fiber: Women with PCOS are at an increased risk of insulin resistance, possibly contributing to elevated blood sugar levels and weight gain.

Consuming high-fiber meals such as fruits, vegetables, whole grains, and legumes may help manage blood sugar levels and increase insulin sensitivity.

Protein: Protein is vital for developing and repairing tissues and may help women with PCOS feel fuller for longer. Lean protein foods like chicken, fish, tofu, and beans are healthy alternatives.

Good Fats: Healthy fats, such as those found in avocados, nuts, seeds, and olive oil, may help increase insulin sensitivity and decrease inflammation.

Micronutrients: Some micronutrients, such as vitamin D and magnesium, may be especially helpful for women with PCOS. The introduction should explain why these nutrients are essential and suggest how to include them in the diet.

Lastly, the introduction highlights the significance of collaborating with a healthcare physician or qualified dietitian to build a specific PCOS diet plan. Although there are broad principles that may be useful for women with PCOS, everyone's nutritional requirements and objectives will be different, and it's crucial to consult with a specialist to ensure that any dietary modifications are safe and successful.

1.1 Understanding PCOS

Understanding PCOS entails understanding what PCOS is, how it affects the body, and the possible health concerns. PCOS is a hormonal illness that affects the ovaries and may produce various symptoms, such as irregular periods, increased hair growth, acne, and weight gain. It is believed that up to 10% of women of reproductive age may have PCOS, making it one of the most frequent hormonal illnesses affecting women.

PCOS is characterized by an imbalance of hormones in the body, notably an excess of androgens (male hormones) and insulin resistance. The specific source of this hormone imbalance is not understood, although genetics and environmental factors are considered to have a role.

The symptoms of PCOS may vary from woman to woman, and not all women with PCOS will have every symptom. Common symptoms include:

- Irregular periods or no periods at all
- Excessive hair growth on the face, chest, or back
- Acne or greasy skin
- Weight gain or difficulty losing weight
- Difficulties getting pregnant
- Dark spots of skin on the neck, groin, or underarms

In addition to these symptoms, women with PCOS are at a greater risk of acquiring certain health issues, such as type 2 diabetes, heart disease, and endometrial cancer. This is why it's crucial for women with PCOS to take action to control their symptoms and lower their risk of serious health concerns.

While there is no cure for PCOS, treatments can help manage symptoms and improve overall health. These treatments may include lifestyle changes such as diet and exercise, medication to regulate periods or reduce androgen levels, and fertility treatments for women who are trying to get pregnant.

Overall, understanding PCOS is important for women diagnosed with the condition or who suspect that they may have it. By learning about the symptoms, causes, and potential health risks of PCOS, women can take steps to manage their symptoms and reduce their risk of associated health problems.

1.2 How Nutrition Can Help Manage PCOS Symptoms

Nutrition has a significant part in treating PCOS symptoms. A good diet may help control hormones, improve insulin sensitivity, and reduce inflammation, all important factors in managing PCOS.

These are several ways that eating might help treat PCOS symptoms:

Regulating insulin levels: Women with PCOS are at an increased risk of insulin resistance, which can lead to high blood sugar levels and weight gain. A diet high in fiber and low in refined carbohydrates can help regulate blood sugar levels and improve insulin sensitivity.

Reducing inflammation: Chronic inflammation is thought to play a role in developing PCOS. A diet with anti-inflammatory foods such as fruits, vegetables, nuts, and seeds may help decrease inflammation.

Enhancing hormonal balance: Some foods, such as omega-3 fatty acids, may help control hormones in people with PCOS. Omega-3s are present in fatty fish, such as salmon and tuna, as well as in walnuts, chia seeds, and flaxseeds.

Managing weight: Weight gain is a common symptom of PCOS, and losing weight can help improve symptoms such as irregular periods and insulin resistance. A diet low in calories and heavy in protein and fiber can help women with PCOS lose weight healthily and sustainably.

Improving fertility: Women with PCOS may have difficulty getting pregnant due to irregular periods and hormonal imbalances. A diet rich in nutrients such as folic acid and iron can help improve fertility in women with PCOS.

It's important to note that there is no one-size-fits-all approach to nutrition for women with PCOS. Every woman is different and may have unique nutritional needs based on her age, weight, and overall health. Working with a registered dietitian can help women with PCOS develop a personalized nutrition plan tailored to their needs and goals.

A healthy and balanced diet can be key in managing PCOS symptoms and improving overall health. By embracing nutrient-rich meals and avoiding processed and high-sugar foods, women with PCOS may take charge of their health and manage their symptoms naturally and effectively.

1.2.1 Control insulin levels

Nutrition may help manage insulin levels in women with PCOS by adopting a fiber-rich diet low in processed carbs. This diet may help lower insulin resistance, a major PCOS symptom.

Insulin resistance develops when the body's cells become less receptive to insulin, a hormone controlling blood sugar levels. This may lead to high blood sugar levels and weight growth, which are prominent signs of PCOS.

These are some ways that eating might help manage insulin levels in people with PCOS:

Consume a balanced diet: A balanced diet that includes a variety of nutrient-rich foods like as fruits, veggies, whole grains, protein, and healthy fats will help manage blood sugar levels and increase insulin sensitivity.

Avoid refined carbs: Refined carbohydrates, such as white bread, spaghetti, and sugary snacks, may increase blood sugar levels and aggravate insulin resistance. Avoiding these meals and selecting whole grains may help manage blood sugar levels and increase insulin sensitivity.

Select high-fiber foods: Meals rich in fiber, like fruits, vegetables, and whole grains, may help manage blood sugar levels and increase insulin sensitivity. Fiber slows down the absorption of carbs in circulation, which helps reduce rises in blood sugar levels.

Incorporate protein in every meal: Protein may help manage blood sugar levels and enhance insulin sensitivity. Eating protein in every meal may help manage blood sugar levels throughout the day.

Minimize added sugars: Added sugars, such as those found in soda, candy, and baked goods, may increase blood sugar levels and aggravate insulin resistance. Limiting added sugars and choosing natural sources of sweetness, such as fruit, can help regulate blood sugar levels and improve insulin sensitivity.

Overall, diet is crucial in treating insulin resistance in women with PCOS. By maintaining a healthy and balanced diet high in fiber and low in refined carbs, women with PCOS may manage blood sugar levels and enhance insulin sensitivity, leading to better overall health and decreased PCOS symptoms.

1.2.2 Decrease inflammation

Nutrition may help lower inflammation in women with PCOS by supporting a diet high in anti-inflammatory foods and low in pro-inflammatory foods. Chronic inflammation is known to have a role in developing PCOS, and lowering inflammation may help control symptoms such as acne, hirsutism, and irregular periods.

Here are some ways that eating might help lower inflammation in people with PCOS:

Consume a diet rich in anti-inflammatory foods: Foods high in antioxidants, vitamins, and minerals may help decrease inflammation. Examples of anti-inflammatory foods include fruits, vegetables, nuts, seeds, fatty fish (such as salmon and tuna), and herbs and spices (such as turmeric and ginger) (such as turmeric and ginger).

Avoid pro-inflammatory meals: Some foods might cause inflammation and aggravate PCOS symptoms. They include processed and fried meals, sugary beverages and snacks, and foods rich in saturated and trans fats.

Incorporate omega-3 fatty acids in the diet: Omega-3 fatty acids have been demonstrated to have anti-inflammatory properties and may help treat PCOS symptoms such as irregular periods and insulin resistance. Omega-3s are present in fatty fish (such as salmon and tuna), walnuts, chia seeds, and flaxseeds.

Reduce alcohol consumption: Alcohol may cause inflammation and aggravate PCOS symptoms. Reducing alcohol intake or eliminating it might help decrease inflammation and improve overall health.

Keep hydrated: Consuming enough water will help flush out toxins from the body and minimize inflammation. Try to drink at least 8-10 glasses of water every day.

It's essential to remember that lowering inflammation is only one part of treating PCOS. A holistic strategy with other lifestyle modifications, such as regular exercise and stress management, is vital for general health and symptom control.

Overall, the diet has a significant role in lowering inflammation in women with PCOS. By adopting a diet high in anti-inflammatory foods and low in pro-inflammatory foods, women with PCOS may control their symptoms and enhance their overall health and well-being.

1.2.3 Enhance hormonal balance

Diet may be crucial in promoting hormonal balance in women with PCOS. Women with PCOS have hormonal imbalances, such as high amounts of androgens (male hormones) and insulin resistance, which may contribute to symptoms such as acne, hirsutism, and irregular periods. A healthy and balanced diet may enhance hormonal balance and lessen these symptoms.

These are some ways that eating might assist in restoring hormonal balance in individuals with PCOS:

Consume a balanced diet: A balanced diet that includes a range of nutrient-rich foods such as fruits, veggies, whole grains, protein, and healthy fats will help manage blood sugar levels and increase insulin sensitivity, which can help lower androgen levels.

Select low-glycemic index (GI) foods: Low-glycemic index absorbed more slowly and induce a slower increase in blood sugar levels, which may help decrease insulin resistance enhance hormonal balance.

Incorporate healthy fats in the diet: Good fats, such as those found in fatty fish, nuts, seeds, and avocado, may assist in restoring hormonal balance by lowering inflammation and supporting the production of hormones.

Avoid processed and refined meals: Processed and refined foods, such as white bread, spaghetti, and sugary snacks, may increase blood sugar levels and aggravate insulin resistance, leading to hormonal imbalances.

Reduce dairy intake: Excessive consumption of dairy products has been associated with higher androgen levels in women. Reducing consumption or adopting dairy replacements such as almond or coconut milk may enhance hormonal balance.

Try taking supplements: Some supplements, such as omega-3 fatty acids, vitamin D, and inositol, have been demonstrated to enhance hormonal balance in women with PCOS.

It's essential to remember that although eating may improve hormonal balance in women with PCOS, it's not a cure. Other lifestyle adjustments, such as regular exercise and stress management, are equally crucial for general health and symptom management.

A healthy and balanced diet may significantly promote hormonal balance in people with PCOS. Women with PCOS may control their symptoms and enhance their overall health and well-being by selecting the proper meals and eliminating processed and refined foods.

1.2.4 Control weight

Nutrition plays a significant part in regulating weight in women with PCOS. Weight control is critical for women with PCOS since excess weight may increase symptoms such as insulin resistance, hormone abnormalities, and inflammation. A nutritious and balanced diet may help control weight and enhance overall health in women with PCOS.

These are some ways that diet might help regulate weight in individuals with PCOS:

Select low-glycemic index (GI) foods: Low-GI foods, such as whole grains, fruits, and vegetables, are absorbed more slowly and produce a slower increase in blood sugar levels, which may help decrease insulin resistance and aid weight reduction.

Incorporate protein in the diet: Protein is vital for weight control since it helps promote fullness and decrease cravings. Select lean protein sources, such as chicken, fish, tofu, and lentils.

Avoid sugary and processed meals: Sugary and processed foods are rich in calories and may lead to weight gain. Avoiding these meals and preferring complete, nutrient-dense foods may help control weight.

Employ portion control: Eating too much, even nutritious foods may lead to weight gain. Exercise portion management by using smaller plates, monitoring meal servings, and being conscious of hunger and fullness signals.

Keep hydrated: Consuming enough water will help decrease cravings and aid weight reduction. Try to drink at least 8-10 glasses of water every day.

It's crucial to remember that although diet might help control weight in women with PCOS, it's not a replacement for regular exercise and other lifestyle adjustments. Frequent physical exercises, such as walking, swimming, or yoga, may also help control weight and improve overall health in women with PCOS.

A healthy and balanced diet may significantly regulate weight in people with PCOS. Women with PCOS may manage their weight and enhance their overall health and well-being by selecting the proper meals, exercising portion control, and keeping hydrated.

The experience of Emily, a lady in her mid-30s who has been diagnosed with PCOS and has been dealing with infertility for some years. Emily has tried several medical procedures and reproductive medicines, but with little result.

Feeling dissatisfied and disillusioned, Emily seeks alternate techniques to enhance her fertility. She goes to a nutritionist specializing in PCOS and fertility, hoping to discover a treatment that would work for her.

The nutritionist works closely with Emily to build a tailored nutrition plan focusing on low-glycemic index meals, lean protein sources, healthy fats, and vital nutrients such as folate, iron, and omega-3 fatty acids. Emily also takes supplements advised by the nutritionist, including inositol, which has been known to boost ovulation and fertility in women with PCOS.

At first, Emily is doubtful about the significance of diet in boosting her fertility. But, after a few weeks of following the dietary plan, she notices some improvements. Her menstrual cycle becomes more regular, and she suffers fewer symptoms of PCOS, such as acne and hair loss.

Throughout the following three months, Emily followed the eating plan and took the supplements advised by the nutritionist. She also adds regular exercise to her schedule, such as yoga and walking.

To her astonishment and excitement, Emily realizes she is pregnant a few months later. She owes her enhanced fertility to the eating regimen and vitamins prescribed by the nutritionist, which helped balance her hormones and improve her ovulation.

Emily's experience demonstrates the strong impact of diet in enhancing fertility in people with

PCOS. Although medical treatments and fertility medicines may be essential in certain situations, a healthy and balanced diet may give a complementary approach to enhancing fertility and raising the chances of pregnancy.

1.3 Essential Nutrients for PCOS

Many crucial nutrients are especially helpful for women with PCOS.

These nutrients help balance hormones, increase insulin sensitivity, decrease inflammation, and support general health and well-being.

Inositol is a kind of sugar alcohol that has been proved to increase insulin sensitivity and stimulate ovulation in women with PCOS. It is found naturally in foods such as citrus fruits, legumes, and whole grains, but supplementation is also available.

Omega-3 fatty acids: Omega-3 fatty acids, present in fatty fish, flaxseed, and chia seeds, may help decrease inflammation and improve hormonal balance in women with PCOS.

Vitamin D: Vitamin D insufficiency is frequent in women with PCOS and has been related to insulin resistance and other health concerns. Vitamin D is present in fatty fish, egg yolks, and fortified meals, although supplements may be required to obtain optimum levels.

Folate: Folate is vital for fetal development and may boost fertility in women with PCOS. It is present in leafy green vegetables, beans, and fortified grains.

Iron deficiency is especially frequent in women with PCOS, particularly those with the excessive monthly flow. Iron-rich foods include red meat, beans, and leafy green vegetables.

Chromium: Chromium is a mineral that may help increase insulin sensitivity and lessen sugar cravings. It is present in broccoli, mushrooms, and whole grains.

Magnesium: Magnesium is vital for hormone control and insulin sensitivity. It is found in leafy green vegetables, nuts, and whole grains.
By integrating these critical nutrients into their diet, women with PCOS may help balance their hormones, increase insulin sensitivity, decrease

inflammation, and promote overall health and well-being. It's crucial to remember that these nutrients are best received through whole meals, although supplements may be required in certain circumstances to attain optimum levels. Women with PCOS should collaborate with a healthcare professional or certified dietitian to build a tailored nutrition plan that meets their needs.

2.0 Getting Started with a PCOS Diet.

2.1 PCOS Diet Recommendations

A PCOS diet should concentrate on nutrient-dense foods that support hormonal balance, increase insulin sensitivity, and minimize inflammation. These are some broad recommendations to follow:

Prioritize whole, unprocessed foods: Select whole grains, fruits, vegetables, lean protein sources, and healthy fats. Avoid processed meals, refined carbs, and sugary drinks.

Examples: quinoa, brown rice, sweet potatoes, berries, leafy greens, nuts and seeds, lean protein sources such as chicken, fish, and tofu, avocado, and olive oil.

Select low-glycemic index foods: Low-glycemic index meals help balance blood sugar and insulin levels, which is helpful for women with PCOS who may be insulin resistant.

Examples: non-starchy vegetables such as broccoli, spinach, and cauliflower, legumes such as chickpeas and lentils, and whole grains such as quinoa and barley.

Concentrate on healthy fats: Good fats such as omega-3 fatty acids may help decrease inflammation and enhance hormone balance.

Examples: fatty fish such as salmon, mackerel, sardines, flaxseeds, chia seeds, walnuts, and avocado.

Include lean protein sources: Lean protein sources may help manage blood sugar and enhance fullness.

Examples: skinless chicken breast, turkey, fish, tofu, and lentils.

Minimize dairy and red meat: Research shows that excessive consumption of dairy and red meat may be connected with a higher risk of PCOS.

Examples: replace dairy with almond or soy milk, and restrict red meat to a few times each week.

Avoid sugary drinks: Sugary beverages such as soda and juice may increase blood sugar and insulin levels.

Examples: consume water, unsweetened tea, or low-sugar drinks.

Be aware of portion sizes: Consuming too much may lead to weight gain, which can aggravate PCOS symptoms.

Examples: use smaller dishes, measure servings, and avoid dining in front of the TV or computer.

By following these tips, women with PCOS may improve their general health and lessen their symptoms. It's crucial to remember that these rules are generic and may need to be tweaked depending on individual requirements and preferences. Women with PCOS should collaborate with a healthcare physician or certified dietitian to develop a dietary plan.

2.2 Meal Planning Strategies

Meal planning may benefit women with PCOS who wish to follow a healthy and balanced diet.

Here are some techniques for good meal planning:

Plan ahead: Spend time each week to plan out your meals and snacks. This will help ensure you have all the necessary items and eliminate last-minute runs to the grocery store or ordering takeout.

Employ a meal planning template: A meal planning template may help you arrange your weekly meals and snacks. You may find free templates online or design your own.

Select a range of foods: Be sure to incorporate a variety of foods from all the major food categories, such as whole grains, fruits, vegetables, lean proteins, and healthy fats. This will assist in ensuring that you are receiving all the nutrients you need.

Balancing macronutrients: Try to balance macronutrients (carbohydrates, protein, and fat) in each meal and snack. This may help manage blood sugar levels and increase fullness.

Contemplate portion proportions: Be conscious of portion sizes and try to fill half of your plate with non-starchy veggies, a quarter with lean protein, and a quarter with whole grain or starchy vegetables.

Meal prep: Prepare certain meals and snacks in advance to save time throughout the week. This might involve chopping veggies, preparing cereals, or marinating lean meats.

Have nutritious snacks on hand: Have healthy snacks such as almonds, fruit, or cut-up veggies easily accessible for when hunger hits between meals.

Ensure to eat meals: Skipping meals might lead to overeating later in the day and produce blood sugar abnormalities. Try to eat three balanced meals and two healthy snacks each day.

Consider your lifestyle: Customize your food plan to your lifestyle and interests. If you are busy throughout the week, try making meals that can be readily reheated or one-pot recipes that take minimal prep work.

Get assistance: Try working with a qualified dietician or joining a support group to help you keep motivated and on track with your food plan.

By following these meal planning guidelines, women with PCOS may ensure they enjoy a nutritious and balanced diet that promotes their health and well-being.

2.2.1 Plan ahead

Preparing ahead for meals may be done by completing several easy steps:

Put aside time: Plan a set period each week to plan your meals and snacks. This might be on a Sunday afternoon or any other day that works best for you.

Build a meal planning template: Download a meal planning template or make your own to help manage your meals and snacks for the week.

Assess your cupboard and refrigerator: Take inventory of what you currently have on hand and include those things in your meal plan. This will help you avoid purchasing unneeded goods at the grocery shop.

Consider your schedule: Consider your schedule for the week and prepare meals that match your lifestyle. For example, if you have a hectic day, prepare meals that take minimal prep time or can be reheated.

Select recipes: Look through cookbooks or internet cooking sources for supper ideas. Pick meals that incorporate a range of foods from all the major food categories.

Create a shopping list: Based on your meal plan, develop a grocery list of all the items you need for the week.

Shop for groceries: Go food shopping and stick to your list. Avoid purchasing items, not on your list or harmful snacks that may entice you.

Prepare in preparation: Prepare certain meals and snacks in advance, such as cutting vegetables or boiling grains, to save time throughout the week.

By planning for meals, you can guarantee that you are eating a nutritious and balanced diet that promotes your health and well-being. This may also help you save time and money by eliminating last-minute treks to the grocery store or ordering takeout.

2.2.2 Meal Planning Template

Utilizing a meal planning template may be great for arranging your meals and snacks for the week. Here are some pointers on how to utilize a meal-planning template effectively:

Pick a template: Many meal planning templates are accessible online, or you may make your own. Search for one that suits your style and tastes.

Plan for all meals and snacks: Your template should contain breakfast, lunch, supper, and snacks for each day of the week.

Incorporate a range of foods: Try to eat various foods from all the various dietary categories, including fruits, vegetables, whole grains, lean protein, and healthy fats.

Consider your schedule: Consider your schedule for the week and prepare meals that match your lifestyle. For example, if you have a hectic day, prepare meals that take minimal prep time or can be simply reheated.

Utilize leftovers: Prepare dishes that can be quickly reheated or reused for leftovers. This may save time and money while decreasing food waste.

Please keep it simple: Don't overcomplicate your food plan with complicated dishes. Adhere to basic meals that are easy to make and enjoy.

Make modifications: Be bold and modify your food plan as required. If you like eating something other than a specific dish, change it for something different.

Utilizing a meal planning template may save time and minimize stress by knowing precisely what you will be eating each day. This may also help you make better food choices and remain on track with your dietary objectives.

2.3 Cooking Tools and Equipment

Kitchen tools and equipment are vital for cooking and creating nutritious meals. Below are some regularly used kitchen utensils and equipment and their uses:

Chef's knife: A sharp, high-quality chef's knife is needed to chop vegetables, fruits, and meats.

Cutting board: A strong cutting board is vital for preserving your blades and providing a safe and hygienic surface for food preparation.

Measuring cups and spoons: Measurement cups and spoons are important for precisely measuring recipe components.

Mixing bowls: Mixing bowls are necessary for blending components for recipes.

Pots and pans: Various pots and pans in various sizes and materials are required for cooking a range of meals.

Wooden spoons and spatulas: Wooden spoons and spatulas are wonderful for stirring and mixing meals without harming non-stick surfaces.

Tongs: Tongs are handy for flipping and rotating meals when cooking.

Grater: A grater is used for shredding cheese, vegetables, and fruits.

Blender or food processor: A blender or food processor is important for producing smoothies, sauces, and purees.

Oven mitts or potholders: Oven mitts or potholders are essential to protect your hands while handling hot pots and pans or when pulling food out of the oven.

Possessing the correct kitchen tools and equipment does cooking and preparing nutritious meals simpler and more fun. Investing in high-quality tools and equipment that will endure and operate effectively over time is crucial.

Chapter Three

3.0 PCOS-Friendly Breakfast Recipes

While controlling PCOS, starting the day with a balanced and healthy breakfast is vital. Here are some PCOS-friendly breakfast dishes to try:

Greek Yogurt Parfait: Layer plain Greek yogurt, fresh berries, and a sprinkling of granola for a protein-rich and fiber-packed breakfast.

Vegetable and Egg Scramble: Sautee chopped veggies such as spinach, mushrooms, and bell peppers in a non-stick skillet, then scramble with 2 eggs for a hearty and healthy breakfast.

Quinoa Breakfast Bowl: Prepare quinoa according to package directions and top with sliced banana, chopped almonds, and a drizzle of honey for a fiber-rich and protein-packed meal.

Avocado Toast: Toast whole grain bread with mashed avocado, a sprinkling of salt and pepper, and a poached or fried egg for a healthy breakfast.

Berry Oatmeal: Boil old-fashioned oats in almond milk and top with fresh berries, chopped almonds, and a drizzle of honey for a fiber-rich and antioxidant-packed breakfast.

Smoothie Bowl: Mix 1 cup of unsweetened almond milk, 1/2 frozen banana, 1/2 cup frozen berries, and one scoop of protein powder for a nutrient-dense and delicious breakfast.

Morning Burrito: Fill a whole wheat tortilla with scrambled eggs, black beans, chopped vegetables, and a sprinkling of cheese for a protein-packed and hearty meal.

Adding a range of nutritious foods and nutrient-dense ingredients, these PCOS-friendly breakfast dishes may help promote hormone balance and general wellness. Speaking with a healthcare practitioner or registered dietitian is crucial to find the optimal meal plan for individual requirements and objectives.

3.0.1 Greek Yogurt Parfait

Greek Yogurt Parfait is a quick and simple breakfast meal that can be adjusted to fit different tastes. Here is a basic recipe to get started:

Ingredients:

- 1 cup plain Greek yogurt
- 1/2 cup fresh berries (such as strawberries, blueberries, or raspberries) (such as strawberries, blueberries, or raspberries)
- 1/4 cup granola
- One teaspoon honey (optional) (optional)

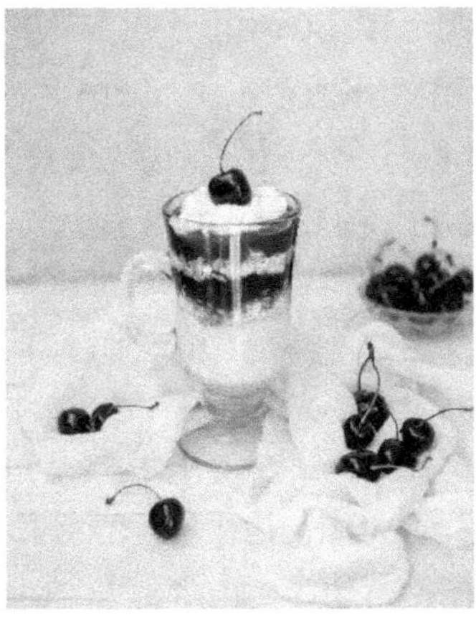

Instructions:

1. In a bowl, mix the Greek yogurt with honey, if using.

2. In a separate bowl, mix the berries.

3. In a serving glass or jar, layer the Greek yogurt, followed by a layer of the mixed berries, and then a layer of granola.

4. Continue the layers until the glass or jar is filled, culminating with a layer of granola on top.

5. Serve warm or refrigerate until ready to eat.

Variations:

- Use unsweetened Greek yogurt and omit the honey for a reduced sugar alternative.
- Replace the granola with chopped nuts or seeds for a lower-carb alternative.
- Add a dab of nut butter for a protein boost.
- Switch out the berries with other fruits, such as sliced banana or mango.

Greek Yogurt Parfait is a flexible breakfast choice that can be readily altered to fit various dietary requirements and tastes. Adding a range of nutrient-dense components may assist in promoting hormone balance and general wellness for persons with PCOS.

3.0.2 Vegetable and Egg Scramble

Vegetable & Egg Scramble is a healthful and substantial breakfast meal that can be easily adjusted to add your favorite veggies and seasonings. Here is a basic recipe to get started:

Ingredients:

- Two eggs
- 1/4 cup chopped bell peppers
- 1/4 cup chopped onion \s1/4 cup diced mushrooms
- 1/4 cup spinach leaves
- Salt and pepper to taste
- One tablespoon of olive oil

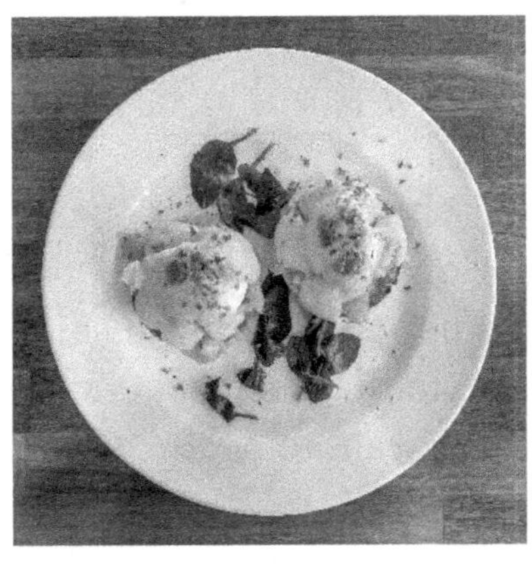

Instructions:

1. In a bowl, mix the eggs with salt and pepper.
2. In a pan over medium heat, add the olive oil and sauté the

diced bell peppers, onion, and mushrooms
until softened, approximately 3-4 minutes.
3. Add the spinach leaves to the pana and heat
until wilted, approximately 1-2 minutes.
4. Dump the whisked eggs into the pan and
scramble until thoroughly cooked,
approximately 2-3 minutes.
5. Serve immediately.

Variations:

- Replace the veggies with your favorites,
such as broccoli, zucchini, or tomatoes.
- Add a sprinkling of cheese for extra taste
and nutrition.
- Serve with avocado or salsa for a healthy
fat boost.
- For added flavor, throw in your favorite
spices, such as cumin or paprika.

Vegetable and Egg Scramble is a protein-rich breakfast choice that delivers a variety of vitamins and minerals from the veggies. It is also a low-carb alternative, making it a perfect choice for persons with PCOS who want to balance their blood sugar levels.

3.0.3 Quinoa Breakfast Bowl:

A Quinoa Breakfast Bowl is a healthful and adaptable breakfast choice that can be adjusted to fit your taste preferences. Here is a basic recipe to get started:

Ingredients:

- 1/2 cup cooked quinoa
- 1/4 cup sliced almonds
- 1/4 cup blueberries
- 1/4 cup sliced strawberries
- 1 tablespoon honey \s1/4 teaspoon cinnamon
- 1/4 cup unsweetened almond milk

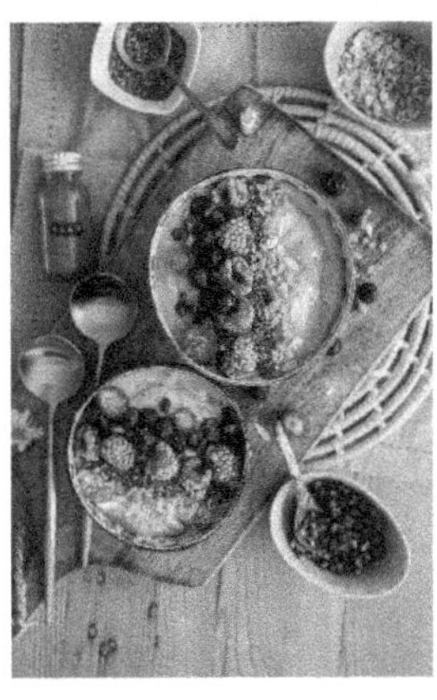

Instructions:

1.   Mix the cooked quinoa, sliced almonds, blueberries, and sliced strawberries in a bowl.
2.   Pour honey over the top and sprinkle with cinnamon.

3. Pour the unsweetened almond milk over the top of the mixture.
4. Serve immediately.

Variations:

- Replace the fruit with your favorites, such as raspberries, blackberries, or bananas.
- Throw in some plain Greek yogurt for additional protein.
- Add maple syrup or agave instead of honey for a vegan alternative.
- Throw in some chia seeds or ground flaxseed for added fiber.

A Quinoa Breakfast Bowl is an excellent choice for people with PCOS since it balances protein, healthy fats, and complex carbs. Quinoa is also a rich source of fiber, which may help to control blood sugar levels and enhance feelings of fullness.

3.0.4 Avocado Toast

Avocado toast is a tasty and easy breakfast choice that can be easily adjusted to meet your tastes. Here is a simple recipe to get started:

Ingredients:

- 1 piece whole grain bread
- 1/2 avocado
- 1/4 teaspoon sea salt
- 1/4 teaspoon black pepper
- 1/4 teaspoon red pepper flakes (optional) (optional)

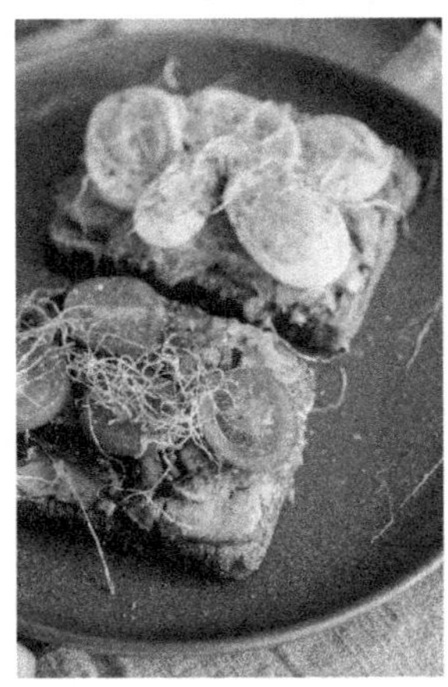

Instructions:

1. Toast the piece of whole grain bread until gently toasted.
2. When the bread is browning, split the avocado and remove the pit.
3. Scoop the avocado flesh into a small dish and mash it with a fork.
4. Distribute the mashed avocado evenly across the bread.
5. Sprinkle sea salt, black pepper, and red pepper flakes (if using) over the top.
6. Serve immediately.

Variations:

- Put a cooked or poached egg on top for extra protein.
- Use gluten-free bread for a gluten-free option.
- Top with sliced tomatoes or cucumber for added flavor and nutrients.
- Top it with crumbled feta cheese or nutritional yeast for extra taste.

Avocado toast is an excellent alternative for persons with PCOS since it contains healthy fats and fiber from avocado and whole-grain bread. The sea salt and black pepper also give a boost of taste without adding additional sodium or calories.

3.0.5 Berry Oatmeal

Berries oatmeal is a tasty and healthy breakfast choice that is simple to make. Here is a simple recipe to get started:

Ingredients:

- 1/2 cup rolled oats

- 1 cup unsweetened almond milk
- 1/2 teaspoon cinnamon
- 1/4 teaspoon vanilla extract
- 1/2 cup mixed berries (fresh or frozen) (fresh or frozen)
- One tablespoon honey or maple syrup (optional) (optional)

Instructions:

1. In a small saucepan, mix the rolled oats and almond milk.
2. Stir the mixture over medium heat, stirring periodically, until the oats have absorbed most of the liquid and are cooked to your desired consistency (approximately 5-7 minutes) (about 5-7 minutes).
3. Mix in the cinnamon and vanilla essence.
4. Add the mixed berries and cook for another 2-3 minutes, until the berries are warmed.
5. If preferred, take the oats from the heat and sweeten them with honey or maple syrup.
6. Serve immediately.

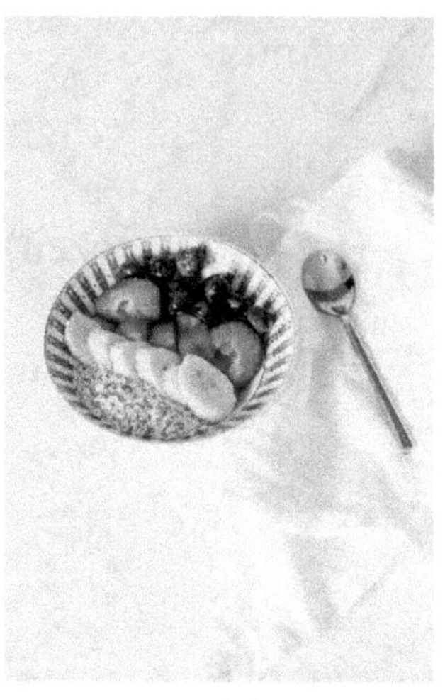

Variations:

- Employ various kinds of milk, such as soy milk or coconut milk, for diverse taste profiles.
- Add sliced bananas or other fruits for extra nutrition and taste.
- For extra protein and healthy fats, sprinkle with chopped nuts, such as almonds or walnuts.
- Mix in a spoonful of chia seeds or powdered flaxseed for additional fiber and omega-3 fatty acids.

Berry oatmeal is a great option for those with PCOS as it provides complex carbohydrates and fiber from oats, antioxidants, and vitamins from mixed berries. The cinnamon and vanilla extract add natural sweetness without excess sugar or calories.

Low-carb breakfast alternatives are a fantastic choice for people with PCOS who want to regulate their blood sugar levels and maintain a healthy weight. Here are a few suggestions for low-carb breakfast options:

Egg Muffins:

Egg muffins are a fantastic make-ahead breakfast option that is low in carbs and strong in protein. Just whisk up some eggs, add chopped veggies (such as bell peppers, spinach, and onions), and bake in a muffin tray for around 20-25 minutes. Prepare a batch at the beginning of the week and reheat them in the morning for a quick and simple breakfast.

Greek Yogurt with Nuts and Berries:

Greek yogurt is an excellent source of protein, and adding nuts and berries to it may make for a satisfying and healthy breakfast. Pick plain Greek yogurt and add your toppings to manage the quantity of sugar in your morning. Consider adding some chopped nuts (such as almonds or walnuts) and a handful of berries for a delightful and low-carb breakfast alternative.

Avocado Toast:

Avocado toast is a popular breakfast choice that is also low in carbs. Pick whole-grain or low-carb bread (like almond flour) and top it with mashed avocado, salt, and pepper. You may also put a poached egg on top for additional protein.

Chia Seed Pudding:

Chia seed pudding is a delightful and low-carb breakfast option that can be cooked beforehand. Just let it rest overnight in the fridge and mix up some chia seeds, almond milk, and a sweetener (such as honey or maple syrup). Top it with fresh fruit or nuts in the morning for extra taste and benefits.

Green Smoothie:

Green smoothies are a terrific way to get veggies and minerals in the morning. Mix together some spinach, kale, or other greens with some low-carb fruits (such as berries or avocado), a source of protein (such as Greek yogurt or protein powder), and some almond milk or coconut water for a tasty and low-carb breakfast option.

These low-carb breakfast alternatives might be a wonderful choice for people with PCOS who want to regulate their blood sugar levels and maintain a healthy weight. These healthy and tasty alternatives can be readily adjusted to match your unique tastes and dietary limitations.

3.1.1 Egg Muffins:

Egg muffins are a terrific low-carb breakfast option that is quick to cook and excellent for meal prep. Here's a recipe to try:

Ingredients:

- Six eggs
- 1/4 cup chopped spinach
- 1/4 cup chopped bell pepper
- 1/4 cup diced onion
- 1/4 cup shredded cheddar cheese
- Salt & pepper, to taste
- Cooking spray

Instructions:

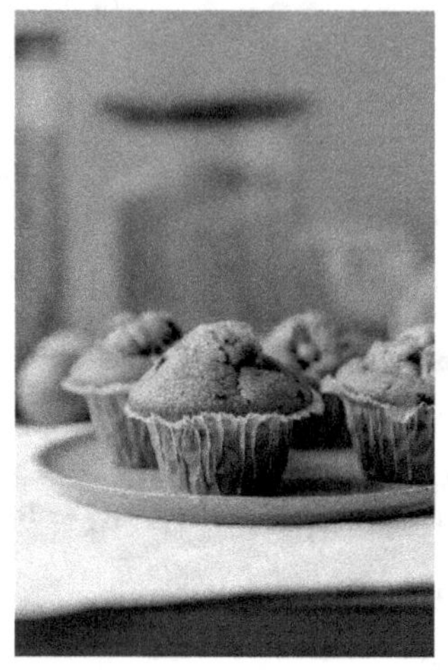

1. Preheat the oven to 350°F.
2. Whisk together the eggs, salt, and pepper in a large bowl until thoroughly blended.
3. Add the chopped spinach, bell pepper, and diced onion to the bowl and toss to incorporate.
4. Spray a muffin tray with cooking spray and equally pour the egg mixture into each muffin cup, filling each approximately 3/4 of the way full.
5. Put shredded cheddar cheese on top of each muffin.
6. Bake for 20-25 mins or until the egg muffins are cooked and slightly browned on top.
7. Let the egg muffins cool briefly before taking them from the pan. Serve hot or keep in the refrigerator for up to 5 days.

Additional variants of egg muffins include adding chopped ham, cooked bacon, or other veggies like mushrooms, tomatoes, or zucchini. You may also experiment with other varieties of cheese or herbs and spices to add extra flavor.

3.1.2 Chia Seed Pudding:

Chia seed pudding is a healthful and substantial breakfast option that is simple to create and adjust to your taste preferences. Here's a recipe to try:

Ingredients:

- 1/4 cup chia seeds
- 1 cup unsweetened almond milk
- 1-2 teaspoons honey or maple syrup (optional) (optional)
- 1/2 teaspoon vanilla extract
- Fresh berries or sliced fruit for topping (optional) (optional)

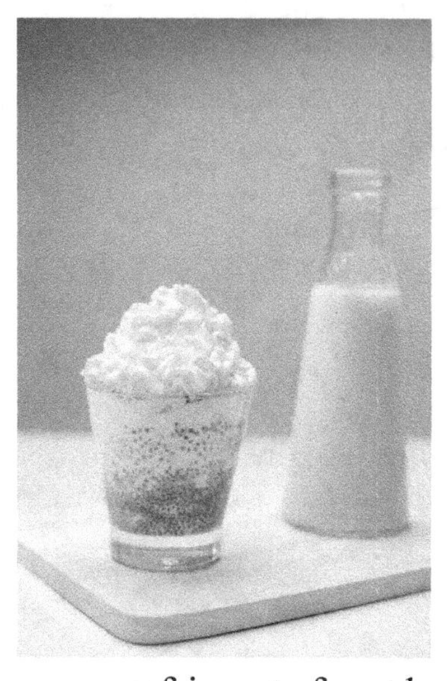

Instructions:

1. In a medium-sized bowl, mix together the chia seeds, almond milk, honey or maple syrup (if using), and vanilla essence until thoroughly incorporated.
2. Cover the bowl with plastic wrap and refrigerate for at least 2 hours, or overnight.
3. After the chia seed pudding has been set, please give it a thorough stir to break up any clumps.
4. Split the pudding into 2-3 dishes or jars, and top with fresh berries or sliced fruit as desired.

Variations of chia seed pudding include adding cocoa powder for a chocolate taste or utilizing various kinds of milk such as coconut milk or oat milk. Add toppings like almonds, shredded coconut, or granola for extra crunch and texture. Try various tastes and toppings to discover your favorite combo!

3.1.3 Green Smoothie

Green smoothies are a healthy and pleasant way to start your day, with fruits and vegetables that give critical vitamins and minerals. Here's an easy recipe to try:

Ingredients:

- 1 banana
- 1 cup fresh spinach
- 1/2 cup frozen mango chunks
- 1/2 cup frozen pineapple chunks
- 1/2 cup unsweetened almond milk
- 1/2 cup plain Greek yogurt
- Optional: 1 tablespoon of honey or maple syrup for sweetness

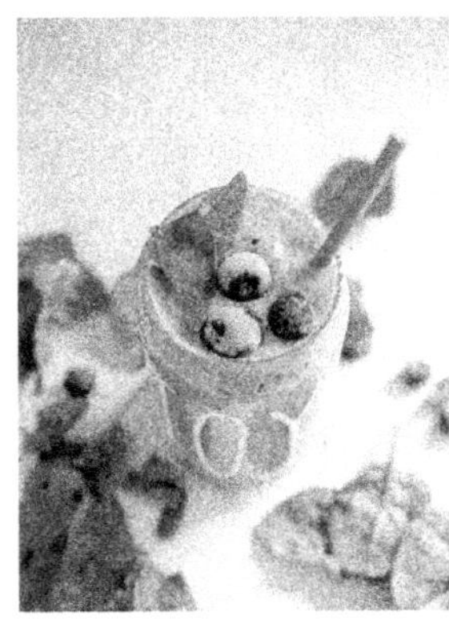

Instructions:

1.   Put all ingredients in a blender and mix until smooth.
2.   If the smoothie is too thick, add additional almond

milk to thin it up to your preferred consistency.

3. Pour the smoothie into a glass and drink immediately.

Variations of green smoothies may include utilizing various greens, such as kale or collard greens, and substituting fruits for your favorites, such as berries or peaches. You may also add protein powder, nut butter, or seeds like chia or flax for more protein and healthy fats. Try various components to get your ideal green smoothie!

3.2 High-Fiber Breakfast Choices

High-fiber breakfast alternatives are wonderful for improving digestive health and keeping you full and content throughout the morning. These are some examples of high-fiber breakfast options:

Overnight oats:

- Combine rolled oats with milk or yogurt.
- Top with fruit, nuts, and seeds.

- Let set in the fridge overnight for a handy and fiber-rich meal.

Whole grain toast with avocado and egg: Toast whole grain bread, top with mashed avocado and a fried or poached egg. Add a sprinkling of salt and pepper for taste.

Smoothie bowl: Mix frozen fruit, yogurt, or milk, and a scoop of protein powder for a thick and creamy smoothie. Sprinkle with fiber-rich toppings like chia seeds, almonds, and fruit for extra texture and nutrition.

High-fiber cereal: Select a cereal with at least 5 grams of fiber per serving and add fresh fruit and nuts for extra crunch and taste.

Greek yogurt parfait: Layer Greek yogurt, fruit, nuts, and granola for a filling and fiber-rich breakfast.

By including high-fiber foods into your morning routine, you may start your day on the right foot and promote a healthy and balanced diet.

3.2.1 Overnight oats:

Overnight oats are a simple and tasty breakfast choice that can be modified with various tastes and additions. Here is a basic recipe for overnight oats:

Ingredients:

- 1/2 cup rolled oats
- 1/2 cup milk (dairy or non-dairy) (dairy or non-dairy)
- 1/4 cup Greek yogurt
- 1-2 tablespoons sweetener (honey, maple syrup, or stevia) (honey, maple syrup, or stevia)
- 1/2 teaspoon vanilla extract
- Pinch of salt

Instructions:

1. Combine the oats, milk, Greek yogurt, sweetener, vanilla extract, and salt in a jar or bowl. Stir to mix.

2. Cover the jar or dish with a cover or plastic wrap and refrigerate overnight or for at least 4 hours.
3. In the morning, sprinkle the oats with your favorite toppings, such as fresh fruit, nuts, seeds, or granola.

Here are some modifications to the basic recipe:

Chocolate peanut butter: Add one tablespoon of chocolate powder and one tablespoon of peanut butter to the basic recipe. Top with sliced banana and chopped peanuts.

Apple cinnamon: Add 1/2 teaspoon cinnamon and 1/2 cup chopped apple to the basic recipe. Top with a dollop of almond butter and a sprinkling of cinnamon.

Blueberry lemon: Add 1/4 cup of blueberries and one teaspoon of lemon zest to the basic recipe. Top with a drizzle of honey and a handful of toasted coconut flakes.

Overnight oats are a flexible and simple breakfast choice that can be cooked ahead of time and adjusted to fit your tastes and preferences. They are also a fantastic source of fiber and protein,

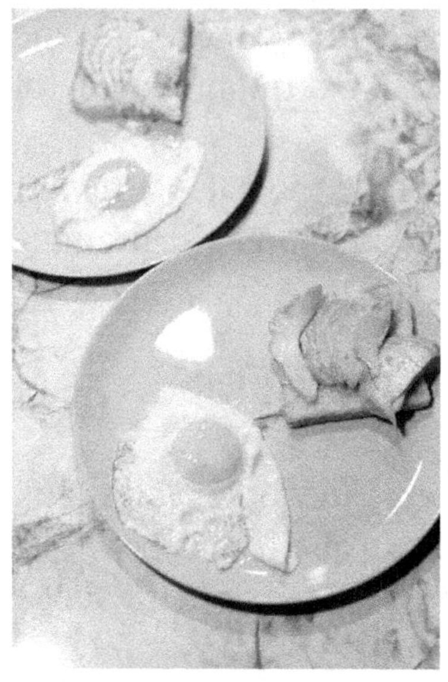

which may help keep you full and pleased throughout the morning.

3.2.2 Whole grain bread with avocado and egg:

Whole grain bread with avocado and egg is a healthy and fulfilling breakfast choice for persons with PCOS. Here is a recipe:

Ingredients:

- One piece of whole-grain bread
- 1/2 ripe avocado
- 1 big egg
- Salt and pepper to taste

Instructions:

1. Toast the bread until it's lightly toasted.

2. While the bread is toasting, mash the avocado in a small dish with a fork.
3. Fry the egg in a non-stick pan until it's done to your preference.
4. Put the mashed avocado on top of the toasted bread.
5. Put the fried egg on top of the avocado.
6. Season with salt and pepper to taste.
7. Serve and enjoy!

This meal is packed in fiber from whole grain bread and healthy fats from the avocado, which helps to increase satiety and manage blood sugar levels. The egg also contains protein, which is needed for creating and repairing structures in the body.

3.2.3 High-fiber cereal

Here is a recipe for a high-fiber cereal:

Ingredients:

- 1/2 cup of whole-grain cereal (e.g., bran flakes, shredded wheat) (e.g., bran flakes, shredded wheat)

- 1/2 cup of fresh berries (e.g., raspberries, blueberries, strawberries) (e.g., raspberries, blueberries, strawberries)
- 1/4 cup of chopped nuts (e.g., almonds, walnuts, pecans) (e.g., almonds, walnuts, pecans)
- 1 cup of unsweetened almond milk or skim milk

Instructions:

1. Mix the whole grain cereal, fresh berries, and chopped almonds in a bowl.
2. Pour the unsweetened almond milk or skim milk over the mixture.
3. Stir well to mix.
4. Let the cereal mixture alone for a few minutes to enable the cereal to soften.

Enjoy your high-fiber cereal!

Note: You may vary the quantity of milk and nuts to your preference and experiment with other varieties of whole-grain cereal and fruit to keep things interesting.

Smoothies and juices may be a terrific way to cram a lot of nutrients into one meal. These are some examples of PCOS-friendly smoothies and juices:

Green Smoothie:

Ingredients:

- 1 cup baby spinach
- 1 cup unsweetened almond milk
- 1/2 frozen banana
- 1/2 cup frozen mango
- One scoop of protein powder
- 1 tsp chia seeds

Instructions:

1. Mix all items until smooth. Enjoy instantly.

Berry Smoothie:

Ingredients:

- 1 cup frozen mixed berries
- 1 cup unsweetened almond milk
- 1/2 frozen banana
- One scoop of protein powder
- 1 tablespoon almond butter

Instructions:

Mix all items until smooth. Enjoy instantly.

Carrot-Apple Juice:

Ingredients:

- Two medium carrots
- 1 medium apple
- 1/2 inch ginger root
- 1/2 lemon

Instructions:

Juice the carrots, apple, and ginger root. Squeeze the juice of 1/2 lemon into the juice and whisk. Enjoy instantly.

Green Juice:

Ingredients:

- 2 cups spinach
- One medium cucumber
- Two medium stalks of celery
- 1/2 lemon

Instructions:

Juice the spinach, cucumber, and celery. Squeeze the juice of 1/2 lemon into the juice and whisk. Enjoy instantly.

Tropical Smoothie:

Ingredients:

- 1/2 cup frozen pineapple
- 1/2 cup frozen mango

- 1/2 frozen banana
- 1 cup unsweetened coconut milk
- One scoop of protein powder

Instructions:

Mix all items until smooth. Enjoy instantly.

While creating smoothies or juices, paying attention to portion proportions is vital, and not overdoing it on the fruit since too much sugar may induce blood sugar spikes. Adding protein and healthy fats to help balance the meal and keep you full is also a good idea.

4.0 PCOS-Friendly Lunch Recipes

4.1 Salads and Bowl Recipes

Salads and bowl recipes are a great way to incorporate vegetables, fruits, whole grains, and proteins into your diet while keeping it interesting and flavorful. Here are some examples of PCOS-friendly salads and bowl recipes:

Mediterranean Quinoa Salad: Cook quinoa according to package directions and mix it with chopped cucumbers, cherry tomatoes, red onion, olives, feta cheese, and fresh parsley. Garnish with olive oil and lemon juice.

Grilled Chicken Salad:
1. Grill chicken breasts and slice them.
2. Stir together greens, cherry tomatoes, cucumber, avocado, and red onion.
3. Top with the sliced chicken and season with olive oil and balsamic vinegar.

Sweet Potato and Black Bean Bowl:

1. Roast sweet potatoes and boil black beans.
2. Combine with brown rice, spinach, avocado, and salsa.
3. Top with a fried egg or grilled chicken for extra protein.

Spinach and Strawberry Salad: Stir together spinach, sliced strawberries, crumbled goat cheese, and chopped walnuts. Dress with a combination of olive oil, balsamic vinegar, and honey.

Greek Salad Bowl:
1. Stir together chopped romaine lettuce, cherry tomatoes, cucumber, red onion, and kalamata olives.
2. Top with feta cheese and grilled chicken or tofu.
3. Dress with olive oil, lemon juice, and dried oregano.

Shrimp and Quinoa Bowl: Prepare quinoa according to package instructions and combine it with grilled shrimp, sliced cucumber, cherry tomatoes, avocado, and cilantro. Dress with a blend of olive oil and lime juice.

Kale Caesar Salad: Stir chopped kale, grilled chicken, cherry tomatoes, and parmesan cheese. Serve with a homemade Caesar dressing from Greek yogurt, lemon juice, garlic, and dijon mustard.

Taco Salad Bowl: Prepare ground turkey or beef with taco seasoning and combine with black beans, chopped lettuce, cherry tomatoes, avocado, and salsa. Cover with grated cheese and serve with brown rice or quinoa.

Asian Chicken Salad: Stir together shredded cabbage, sliced carrots, red pepper, and sliced grilled chicken. Garnish with sesame oil, rice vinegar, soy sauce, and honey.

Quinoa & Roasted Vegetable Bowl: Roast your favorite veggies, such as broccoli, carrots, and bell peppers, then combine them with cooked quinoa. Top with crumbled feta cheese and season with olive oil, lemon juice, and Dijon mustard.

4.1.1 Mediterranean Quinoa Salad

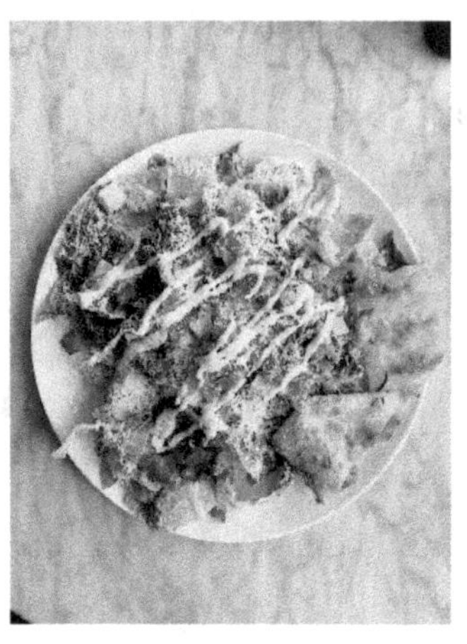

Mediterranean Quinoa Salad is a wonderful and healthful alternative for lunch or supper. Here's a recipe for it:

Ingredients:

- 1 cup quinoa
- One can of chickpeas, drained and rinsed
- 1/2 cup diced cucumber
- 1/2 cup cherry tomatoes, halved
- 1/4 cup chopped red onion
- 1/4 cup chopped fresh parsley
- 1/4 cup crumbled feta cheese
- Two tablespoons of olive oil
- Two teaspoons of red wine vinegar
- One tablespoon of lemon juice
- One clove of garlic, minced
- Salt and pepper to taste

Instructions:

1. Rinse the quinoa under running water and set it in a saucepan with 2 cups of water. Bring to a boil, then decrease heat and let it simmer for 15-20 minutes until the water is absorbed and the quinoa is soft.
2. After cooking the quinoa, please remove it from the heat and cool it to room temperature.
3. Add chickpeas, cucumber, cherry tomatoes, red onion, parsley, and feta cheese in a large mixing basin.
4. Mix the olive oil, red wine vinegar, lemon juice, garlic, salt, and pepper in a small bowl.
5. Add the cooked quinoa to the mixing dish with the veggies and toss to incorporate.
6. Pour the dressing over the salad and toss it again to cover everything evenly.
7. Serve immediately or refrigerate until ready to serve.

This meal is packed with fiber and protein because of the quinoa and chickpeas while adding fresh veggies and healthy fats from the olive oil and feta cheese.

4.1.2 Grilled Chicken Salad

Here is a recipe for Grilled Chicken Salad:

Ingredients:

- Two boneless, skinless chicken breasts
- 1/4 cup olive oil
- Two cloves garlic, minced
- 1 tsp dried oregano
- Salt with black pepper
- 6 cups mixed greens
- 1 cup cherry tomatoes, halved
- 1/2 cup chopped red onion
- 1/4 cup crumbled feta cheese
- 1/4 cup sliced kalamata olives
- Lemon wedges for serving

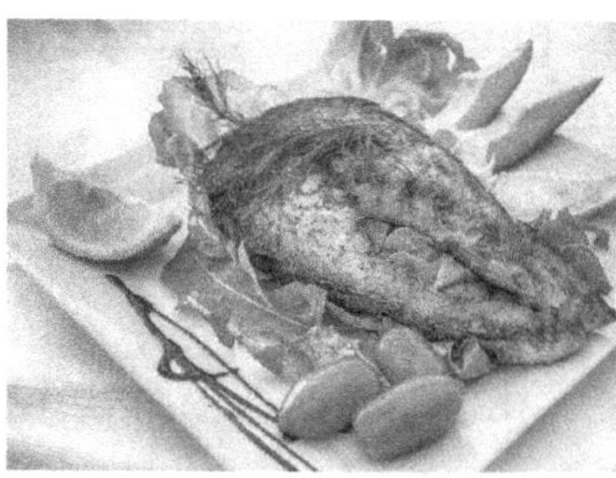

Instructions:

1.   Preheat the grill to medium-high heat.

2. Mix olive oil, garlic, oregano, salt, and pepper in a small bowl.
3. Coat chicken breasts with the oil mixture and carefully coat them evenly.
4. Put chicken on the grill and cook for 6-8 minutes on each side or until cooked.
5. Let chicken rest for 5 minutes before chopping it into thin pieces.
6. Add mixed greens, cherry tomatoes, red onion, feta cheese, and kalamata olives in a large bowl.
7. Top the salad with the sliced chicken.
8. Serve with lemon slices on the side.

This grilled chicken salad is tasty and filled with nutrients that may aid patients with PCOS. The mixed greens give a range of vitamins and minerals, while the cherry tomatoes and red onions contribute antioxidants.

The grilled chicken is an excellent source of protein, which may help manage insulin levels, while the feta cheese and olives give healthy fats. Moreover, lemon wedges might aid in improving digestion and promoting immunity.

4.1.3 Sweet Potato with Black Bean Bowl

Sweet Potato and Black Bean Bowl Recipe:

Ingredients:

- One big sweet potato, peeled and chopped
- 1 can black beans, washed and drained
- One red bell pepper, sliced
- 1 avocado, sliced
- 1/4 cup chopped cilantro
- 1 tablespoon olive oil
- 1 tablespoon chili powder
- 1 teaspoon ground cumin
- Salt and pepper to taste
- Cooked quinoa (optional) (optional)

Directions:

1. Preheat the oven to 425°F. Line a baking sheet with parchment paper.

2. Combine sweet potato, chili powder, cumin, olive oil, salt, and pepper in a bowl. Put the sweet potatoes on the baking sheet and bake for 20-25 minutes or until cooked.

3. In a separate dish, stir together black beans, red bell pepper, cilantro, salt, and pepper.

To construct the bowl:
1. Distribute cooked quinoa (if using) across four bowls.
2. Cover with roasted sweet potato and black bean combination.
3. Add sliced avocado and additional cilantro for garnish.

Note: This meal is full of fiber, protein, and healthy fats. Sweet potato delivers complex carbs that may help control blood sugar levels, while black beans are an excellent source of protein and fiber. The avocado gives healthy fats, while the red bell pepper adds vitamins and antioxidants. Using quinoa as a basis might offer extra fiber and protein to the meal.

4.1.4 Spinach and Strawberry Salad

Spinach and Strawberries Salad is a tasty and healthful salad that is excellent for a light lunch or supper. Here are some recipe ideas:

Spinach & Strawberry Salad with Balsamic Vinaigrette:

Ingredients: baby spinach, fresh strawberries, feta cheese, sliced almonds, balsamic vinegar, olive oil, Dijon mustard, honey, salt, and black pepper.

Directions: In a large bowl, whisk together balsamic vinegar, olive oil, Dijon mustard, honey, salt, and black pepper. Add baby spinach, sliced strawberries, crumbled feta cheese, and sliced almonds to the bowl and toss to combine.

Spinach and Strawberry Salad with Grilled Chicken:

Ingredients: baby spinach, fresh strawberries, grilled chicken breast, crumbled goat cheese, sliced almonds, red onion, balsamic vinegar, olive oil, Dijon mustard, honey, salt, and black pepper.

Directions:
1. Mix balsamic vinegar, olive oil, Dijon mustard, honey, salt, and black pepper in a large bowl.
2. Add baby spinach, sliced strawberries, crumbled goat cheese, sliced almonds, and

thinly sliced red onion to the bowl and blend.
3. Top with sliced grilled chicken breast.

Spinach and Strawberry Salad with Poppy Seed Dressing:

Ingredients: baby spinach, fresh strawberries, red onion, crumbled feta cheese, sliced almonds, plain Greek yogurt, honey, white wine vinegar, poppy seeds, salt, and black pepper.

Directions:
1. In a small bowl, stir together Greek yogurt, honey, white wine vinegar, poppy seeds, salt, and black pepper.
2. Add baby spinach, sliced strawberries, thinly sliced red onion, crumbled feta cheese, and sliced almonds in a large bowl.
3. Pour the poppy seed dressing over the salad and toss to mix.

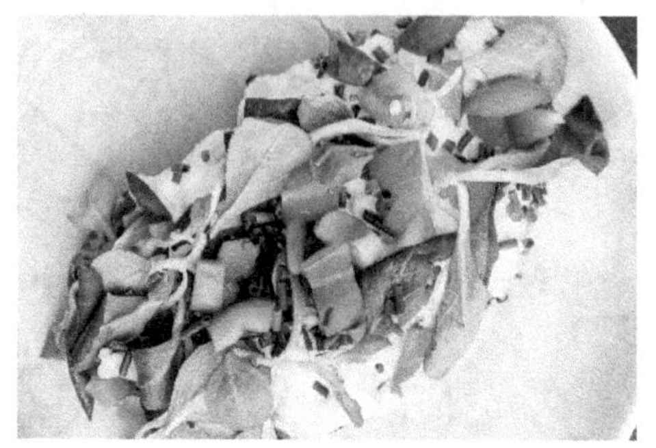

4.1.5 Greek Salad Bowl:

Here's a recipe for a Greek Salad Bowl:

Ingredients:

- 2 cups cooked quinoa
- 1/2 cup crumbled feta cheese
- 1/2 cup sliced cherry tomatoes
- 1/2 cup chopped cucumbers
- 1/2 cup minced red onion
- 1/4 cup chopped kalamata olives
- 1/4 cup chopped fresh parsley
- 1/4 cup chopped fresh mint
- Two teaspoons of lemon juice
- Two tablespoons extra-virgin olive oil
- Salt and pepper to taste

Instructions:

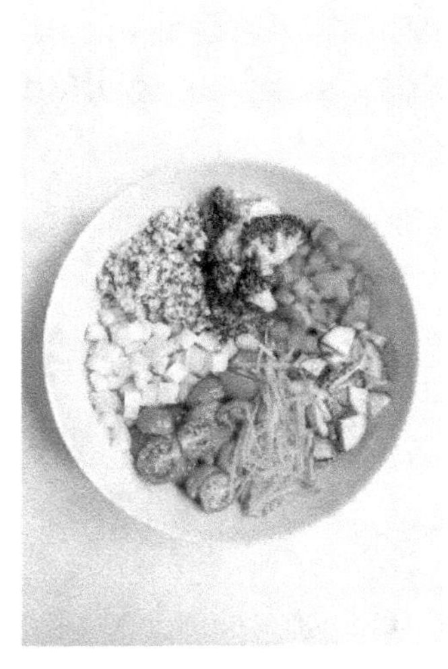

1. Combine the cooked quinoa, crumbled feta cheese, cherry tomatoes, cucumbers, red onion, kalamata olives, parsley, and mint in a large mixing bowl.
2. In a small bowl, mix the lemon juice and olive oil. Pour the dressing over the quinoa salad and toss to coat.
3. Season the salad with salt and pepper to taste.
4. Split the salad into separate dishes and serve immediately.

This Greek Salad Bowl is a nutritious and tasty supper choice filled with nutrients. Quinoa is an excellent plant-based protein and fiber source, while veggies and herbs contribute vitamins and minerals. Feta cheese with kalamata olives delivers a dose of healthy fats.

This salad may be adjusted by adding or replacing different vegetables or meats, such as grilled chicken or chickpeas.

4.1.6 Asian Chicken Salad

Here's a recipe for Asian Chicken Salad:

Ingredients:

- 1 pound boneless, skinless chicken breast
- 1/4 cup soy sauce
- 2 tablespoon rice vinegar
- 2 tablespoon honey
- 1 tablespoon sesame oil
- Two garlic cloves minced
- 1 tablespoon grated fresh ginger
- 4 cups mixed greens
- One red bell pepper, thinly sliced
- 1/2 cup shredded carrots
- 1/2 cup sliced cucumber
- 1/2 cup chopped cilantro
- 1/4 cup chopped scallions
- 1/4 cup chopped peanuts
- Lime wedges for serving

Instructions:

1. Preheat the grill to medium-high heat. Mix the soy sauce, rice vinegar, honey, sesame oil, garlic, and ginger in a small bowl.

2. Put the chicken in a big reseal able bag and pour half of the marinade over it. Close the bag and massage the chicken to coat evenly. Let it marinate for at least 30 minutes.

3. Grill the chicken for 5-6 minutes on each side or until cooked. Let it sit for 5 minutes before slicing.

4. Arrange the salad by dividing the mixed greens into four bowls. Garnish each dish with sliced chicken, red bell pepper, shredded carrots, sliced cucumber, cilantro, scallions, and chopped peanuts.

5. Pour the leftover marinade over the salad or serve it on the side with lime wedges.

Enjoy your tasty and healthful Asian Chicken Salad!

4.1.7 Taco Salad Bowl

Here is a recipe for a taco salad bowl:

Ingredients:

- 1 pound ground beef
- One tablespoon of olive oil
- 1/2 cup chopped onion
- 2 cloves garlic, minced
- One tablespoon of chili powder
- One teaspoon cumin
- 1/2 teaspoon smoked paprika
- 1/2 teaspoon salt
- 1/4 teaspoon black pepper
- 1/4 cup tomato sauce
- One can (15 oz) of black beans, drained and rinsed
- 1 cup corn kernels
- 1/2 cup chopped fresh cilantro
- One head romaine lettuce, chopped \s1 avocado, diced
- 1/2 cup shredded cheddar cheese
- 1/4 cup salsa

- 1/4 cup sour cream
- Lime wedges for serving

Instructions:

1. Heat olive oil in a large pan over medium heat. Add the onion and garlic and simmer for 2-3 minutes, until softened.

2. Add the ground beef, chili powder, cumin, smoked paprika, salt, and black pepper. Sauté, occasionally tossing, until the steak is browned and cooked through, approximately 10-12 minutes.

3. Add the tomato sauce, black beans, and corn to the skillet. Stir to incorporate and simmer for 2-3 minutes until cooked through.

4. Take the pan from the heat and mix in the cilantro.

To construct the salad bowls, divide the chopped lettuce among four bowls. Cover each bowl with

the meat and bean mixture, chopped avocado, shredded cheese, salsa, and sour cream.
Serve with lime wedges for squeezing over the top.

This taco salad bowl is a terrific nutritious and full supper alternative. It offers lean protein from ground beef, fiber from black beans and corn, healthy fats from the avocado, and lots of vitamins and minerals from the romaine lettuce and cilantro. Additionally, it's simple to tailor to your preference by adding or deleting components as needed.

4.2 Sandwiches and Wraps

Sandwiches and wraps are popular lunch choices that may be delicious and healthful. They provide a practical method to incorporate various components into a compact meal that can be eaten on the move. These are some examples of sandwich and wrap recipes:

Turkey and Avocado Wrap: Spread a whole-wheat wrap with mashed avocado, layer with turkey slices, sliced tomatoes, shredded lettuce, and a drizzle of balsamic vinegar.

Veggie Hummus Sandwich: Spread whole-grain bread with hummus and top with sliced cucumbers, bell peppers, shredded carrots, and sprouts.

Grilled Chicken Panini: Layer sliced grilled chicken breast, roasted red peppers, fresh basil leaves, and mozzarella cheese between two slices of whole-grain bread. Grill until the cheese is melted and the bread is toasted.

Egg Salad Sandwich: Combine hard-boiled eggs with Greek yogurt, sliced celery, chopped onions, and a squeeze of lemon juice. Spread over whole-grain bread and top with lettuce leaves.

Tuna Salad Wrap: Combine canned tuna with Greek yogurt, sliced celery, chopped pickles, and a splash of lemon juice. Spread on a whole-wheat wrap and add shredded carrots and sliced cucumber.

BLT Wrap: Spread a whole-grain wrap with mashed avocado, cover with crispy bacon, sliced tomatoes, shredded lettuce, and a sprinkle of balsamic vinegar.

Grilled Vegetable Wrap: Grill sliced eggplant, zucchini, red peppers, and portobello mushrooms. Put on a whole-grain wrap and top with crumbled feta cheese and a drizzle of balsamic glaze.

Falafel Wrap: Fill a whole-grain wrap with baked falafel balls, sliced cucumbers, shredded lettuce, chopped tomatoes, and a dab of tzatziki sauce.

Caprese Panini: Put sliced tomatoes, fresh basil leaves, and mozzarella cheese between two pieces of whole-grain bread. Grill until the cheese is melted and the bread is toasted. Drizzle with balsamic glaze.

Grilled Chicken Caesar Wrap: Grill-sliced chicken breast served on a whole-wheat wrap with shredded romaine lettuce, chopped tomatoes, grated Parmesan cheese, and Caesar dressing.

4.2.1 Turkey and Avocado Wrap:

Here is a recipe for Turkey and Avocado Wrap:

Ingredients:

- One big tortilla wrap
- 2-3 slices of roasted turkey breast
- 1/4 avocado, mashed
- 1/4 cup sliced tomatoes
- 1/4 cup sliced cucumber
- 1/4 cup shredded lettuce
- One tablespoon of plain Greek yogurt
- 1/2 teaspoon Dijon mustard
- Salt and pepper to taste

Directions:

1. Put the tortilla flat on a clean surface.

2. Put the mashed avocado in the Middle of the tortilla.

3. Put the turkey, sliced tomatoes, sliced cucumber, and shredded lettuce on top of the avocado.
4. Mix the Greek yogurt, Dijon mustard, salt, and pepper in a small bowl until thoroughly blended.

5. Pour the sauce over the top of the turkey and veggies.

6. Fold the edges of the tortilla inward, then roll up firmly from the bottom to the top.

7. Split the wrap in half and serve.

This wrap is packed with protein from the turkey and Greek yogurt, healthy fats from the avocado, and fiber from the veggies. It might be a terrific alternative for a fast and simple lunch on the go.

4.2.2 Grilled Chicken Panini

A grilled Chicken Panini is a tasty and easy-to-make sandwich that is excellent for a fast lunch or supper. Here is a recipe for Grilled Chicken Panini:

Ingredients:

- Two boneless, skinless chicken breasts
- 1/4 cup olive oil
- Two cloves garlic, minced
- Salt and pepper to taste
- One big red bell pepper, cut \s1/2 red onion, sliced
- 4 slices provolone cheese
- Four ciabatta slices of bread split in half
- Two tablespoons mayonnaise
- Two teaspoons of Dijon mustard
- One tablespoon honey
- One tablespoon of balsamic vinegar
- 2 cups baby arugula

Instructions:

1. Prepare a grill or grill pan to medium-high heat.

2. Mix the olive oil, garlic, salt, and pepper in a small bowl. Brush the chicken breasts with the mixture.

3. Grill the chicken for 5-6 minutes on each side or until cooked. Remove

from heat and allow rest for 5 minutes, then slice into thin strips.

4. In a large pan over medium heat, sauté the red bell pepper and red onion until soft, approximately 5-7 minutes.

5. Mix the mayonnaise, Dijon mustard, honey, and balsamic vinegar in a small bowl.

To construct the sandwiches:

1. Apply the mayonnaise mixture on the bottom half of each ciabatta bun.
2. Top with sliced chicken, sautéed veggies, and a piece of provolone cheese.
3. Top with baby arugula and the other half of the ciabatta bread.

Heat a panini press or grill pan over medium heat. Put the sandwiches on the panini press or grill pan and heat for 3-4 minutes, or until the bread is crispy and the cheese is melted.

Enjoy your wonderful Grilled Chicken Panini!

4.2.3 BLT Wrap

Here is a recipe for a great and nutritious BLT wrap:

Ingredients:

- One whole wheat tortilla wrap
- 2-3 pieces of turkey bacon
- One small tomato cut
- 1-2 big lettuce leaves
- One tablespoon mayonnaise
- Salt and pepper to taste

Instructions:

1. Sauté the turkey bacon in a pan over medium heat until it's crispy, then put it aside on a paper towel to drain any extra grease.

2. Preheat the tortilla in the pan for a few seconds on each side.

3. Pour mayonnaise evenly over the tortilla, leaving approximately an inch from the borders.

4. Put the lettuce leaves on top of the mayonnaise.

5. Put the sliced tomato on top of the lettuce.

6. Cut the bacon into tiny pieces and sprinkle them over the tomato.

7. Season with salt and pepper to taste.

8. Roll the wrap firmly, tucking in the edges to prevent the contents from spilling out.

9. Split the wrap in half and serve.

This wrap is a tasty and healthy alternative to a traditional BLT sandwich, including whole wheat tortilla and turkey bacon. You may also add veggies, such as cucumber or avocado, to improve the nutritious value. Enjoy!

4.2.4 Falafel Wrap

Falafel wraps are a popular Middle Eastern meal that may be readily produced at home. They are a nutritious and tasty alternative for a fast lunch or supper.

Here's a recipe for falafel wraps:

Ingredients:

- One can of chickpeas, drained and rinsed
- 1/2 cup of fresh parsley
- 1/2 cup of fresh cilantro
- 1/2 onion, chopped
- Three garlic cloves minced
- 2 tablespoons of flour
- One teaspoon of ground cumin
- One teaspoon of ground coriander
- 1/4 teaspoon of cayenne pepper
- Salt and pepper to taste
- Four whole wheat tortillas
- 1 cup of chopped lettuce
- 1/2 cup of chopped tomatoes
- 1/2 cup of diced cucumber
- 1/4 cup of crumbled feta cheese
- 1/4 cup of hummus

- 1/4 cup of tzatziki sauce

Instructions:

1. Add chickpeas, parsley, cilantro, onion, garlic, flour, cumin, coriander, cayenne pepper, salt, and pepper in a food processor. Pulse until thoroughly blended and somewhat chunky.

2. Shape the mixture into tiny patties approximately 2 inches in diameter.

3. Heat a large pan over medium heat and lightly coat with cooking spray.

4. Sauté the patties in the skillet until browned on both sides, approximately 2-3 minutes on each side.

5. Warm up the tortillas in the microwave or on a grill.

6. Put hummus in the Middle of each tortilla.

7. Put the lettuce, tomatoes, and cucumber on top of the hummus.

8. Add the falafel patties and top with feta cheese.

9. Drizzle with tzatziki sauce.

10. Fold the tortilla to make a wrap and serve.

This recipe produces four servings.

4.3 Soups & Stews

Soups and stews are warm and comforting meals that may be filled with nutrition and taste. They are particularly adaptable since they can be cooked large amounts and refrigerated for simple reheating and leftovers. Here are some examples of recipes for soups and stews:

Chicken Noodle Soup: This classic soup is a favorite for many and is easy to make. Start by cooking chicken breast in chicken broth until it is cooked through. Take the chicken from the soup and shred it. Add chopped carrots, celery, and onion to the broth and simmer until the vegetables are tender. Put the shredded chicken back into the broth with cooked noodles, and season with salt and pepper to taste.

Lentil Soup: Lentil soup is a healthy, nourishing, vegetarian-friendly alternative. Start by sautéing chopped onion, celery, and carrots in olive oil. Add lentils, vegetable broth, and canned chopped tomatoes to the saucepan and heat to a boil. Sauté until the lentils are soft, then add chopped kale or spinach for some added nourishment.

Beef Stew: Beef stew is a hearty and comforting option for a cold day. Start by searing beef stew meat in a Dutch oven until it is browned on both sides. Take the meat from the saucepan and sauté chopped onions and garlic until soft. Add chopped carrots, celery, beef stock, canned diced tomatoes, and seared meat into the saucepan. Cook until the meat is soft and the veggies are cooked through. Serve with fresh bread for dipping.

Tomato Soup: Tomato soup is a traditional choice that is simple to cook and flavorful. Start by sautéing chopped onions and garlic in a saucepan until soft. Add canned tomatoes, vegetable broth, and a splash of cream to the saucepan and cook until the flavors are blended. Use an immersion blender to puree the soup until it is smooth, and season with salt and pepper to taste.

Chili: Chili is a meaty, spicy, excellent meal for a comfortable night. Start by cooking ground beef or turkey in a saucepan until browned. Take the meat from the saucepan and sauté chopped onions and garlic until soft. Add canned kidney beans, diced tomatoes, tomato sauce, chili powder, and cooked beef to the saucepan. Cook until the flavors are blended, and season with salt and pepper to suit.

These are only a few examples of recipes for soups and stews, but there are countless alternatives to explore. With the right ingredients and flavors, soups and stews may be a nutritious and tasty supper choice for any occasion.

4.3.1 Chicken Noodle Soup:

Chicken noodle soup is a traditional comfort dish that is full and nourishing. Here's a recipe to make homemade chicken noodle soup:

Ingredients:

- 1 pound boneless, skinless chicken breasts
- 8 cups chicken broth
- 3 medium carrots, peeled and chopped
- 3 stalks celery, chopped
- 1 medium onion, chopped
- 3 cloves garlic, minced
- One teaspoon of dried thyme
- 1 bay leaf
- 8 ounces egg noodles
- Salt and pepper to taste

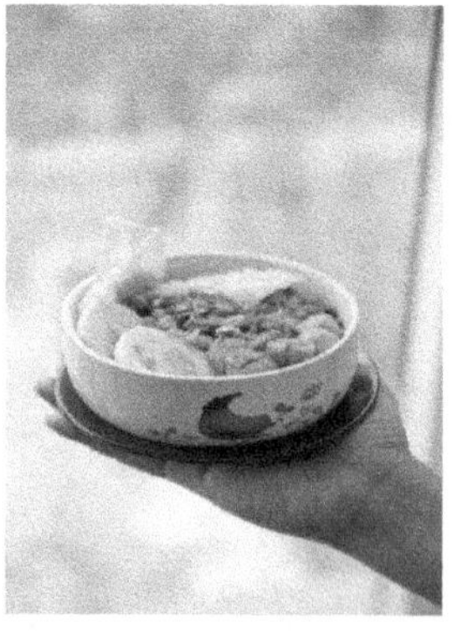

Instructions:

1.   Begin by cooking the chicken in a big saucepan of boiling water for approximately 20 minutes until thoroughly done. Take

the chicken from the pot and put it aside to cool. After it has cooled, shred it into little pieces.

2. In the same saucepan, heat some oil over medium heat. Add the chopped onions, carrots, celery, and sauté until they become soft, which will take approximately 5 minutes.

3. Add the minced garlic, thyme, bay leaf, and chicken broth to the saucepan. Bring the mixture to a boil, then decrease the heat to low and let it simmer for approximately 20 minutes.

4. Add the shredded chicken to the stew and let it simmer for another 5 minutes.

5. In a separate pot, cook the egg noodles according to the package directions.

6. After the noodles are done, add them to the saucepan with the broth and

chicken. Simmer for another 5 minutes.

7. Add salt and pepper to taste.

Your homemade chicken noodle soup is now ready to serve. Enjoy!

4.3.2 Lentil Soup

Lentil soup is a warm and healthful soup that is excellent for a chilly winter day. It is a vegetarian soup rich in protein, fiber, and minerals. Here's a recipe for lentil soup:

Ingredients:

- One tablespoon of olive oil
- One onion, chopped
- 2 carrots, chopped
- 2 celery stalks, chopped
- 2 garlic cloves, minced
- One teaspoon of ground cumin
- 1/2 teaspoon ground coriander
- 1/2 teaspoon smoked paprika
- 1/4 teaspoon ground turmeric

- 1/4 teaspoon cayenne pepper (optional) (optional)
- One bay leaf
- 1 cup dry lentils, washed and drained
- 4 cups vegetable broth \s1 can (14.5 oz) (14.5 oz) chopped tomatoes
- Salt and pepper to taste
- Chopped fresh parsley for garnish

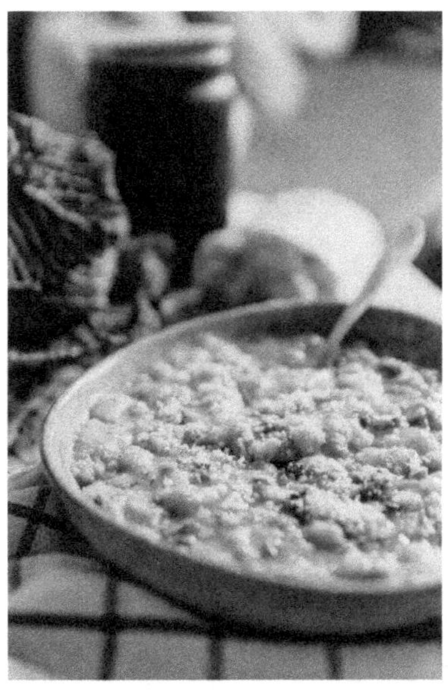

Directions:

1.   Heat the olive oil in a big saucepan over medium heat. Add the onion, carrots, and celery, and simmer for 5-7 minutes, turning periodically, until the veggies are soft.

2.   Add the garlic, cumin, coriander, smoked paprika, turmeric, and cayenne pepper (if using), and simmer for another minute, frequently stirring, until aromatic.

3. Add the bay leaf, lentils, vegetable broth, and chopped tomatoes, and bring the soup to a boil.

4. Lower the heat, cover the pot, and simmer the soup for 30-40 minutes or until the lentils are cooked.

5. Season the soup with salt and pepper to taste.

6. Spoon the soup into dishes, then top with chopped fresh parsley.

Enjoy your healthy and tasty lentil soup!

4.3.3 Beef Stew

Beef stew is a traditional comfort dish that may be produced at home. Here is a recipe for beef stew that feeds six:

Ingredients:

- 2 pounds of beef stew meat, sliced into 1-inch chunks

- Two tablespoons of olive oil
- 2 tablespoons all-purpose flour
- 2 cups beef broth
- 1 onion, chopped \s4 cloves garlic, minced
- Four carrots, peeled and sliced
- Four stalks of celery cut
- One can of chopped tomatoes (14.5 ounces) (14.5 ounces)
- Two tablespoons dried thyme
- Two tablespoons of dried rosemary
- Salt & pepper, to taste

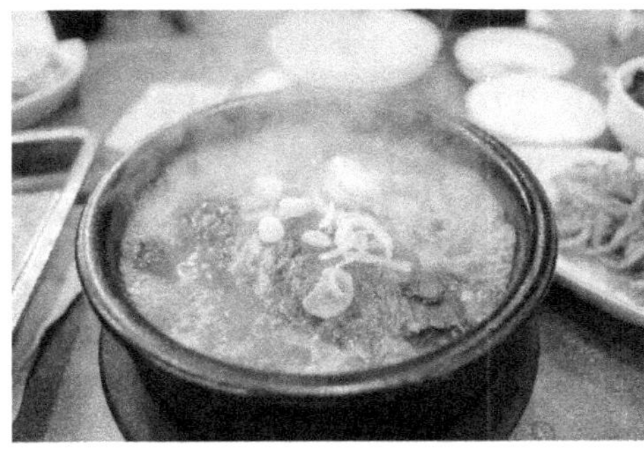

Instructions:

1.   Prepare a large saucepan or Dutch oven over medium-high heat. Add olive oil and beef stew meat. Brown, the meat on both sides, then remove from the saucepan and set aside.

2. Add onions and garlic to the saucepan and sauté for a few minutes until the onions are transparent.

3. Add flour to the saucepan and swirl to coat the onions and garlic. Cook for 1-2 minutes.

4. Gradually pour in beef broth, frequently stirring to avoid lumps. Bring to a boil.

5. Return the meat to the saucepan along with carrots, celery, diced tomatoes, thyme, rosemary, salt, and pepper. Stir to mix.

6. Lower heat to low and simmer for 1-2 hours until meat is tender and veggies are cooked through.

7. Serve hot, and enjoy your excellent beef stew!

4.3.4 Tomato Soup

Tomato soup is a popular comfort dish that may be cooked with fresh or tinned tomatoes. Here's an easy recipe for preparing tomato soup:

Ingredients:

- Four cups of diced fresh tomatoes or 28 oz. canned tomatoes
- 1 cup of chicken or vegetarian broth
- 1/4 cup of unsalted butter
- 1 diced onion
- 1 tablespoon of minced garlic
- One tablespoon of sugar
- One tablespoon of tomato paste
- 1/4 cup of chopped fresh basil leaves or one teaspoon of dried basil
- 1/2 cup of heavy cream
- Salt and pepper to taste

Instructions:

1. Melt the butter in a big saucepan over medium heat. Add the chopped onion and heat until it turns transparent.

2. Add the garlic and simmer for another minute.

3. Add the diced tomatoes, chicken or vegetable broth, sugar, and tomato paste. Stir to mix and bring to a boil.

4. Lower the heat to low and let the mixture simmer for approximately 20 minutes or until the tomatoes have broken down.

5. Take the saucepan from the heat and allow the mixture to cool for a few minutes.

6. Use an immersion blender to puree the ingredients until it is smooth. If you don't have an immersion blender, you may transfer the mixture to a blender and blend in batches.

7. Bring the saucepan to the heat and add the chopped or dried basil leaves. Simmer for a couple more minutes.

8. Whisk in the heavy cream and season with salt and pepper to taste.

9. Serve the tomato soup hot with some crusty bread or a grilled cheese sandwich. You may also garnish

with some fresh basil leaves or croutons.

Please write in English (US) language.
Chili is a traditional, hearty, comforting meal that is great for chilly times. It is often cooked with ground beef, beans, tomatoes, and spices. These are a few different recipes for chili:

Classic Beef Chili:

- One lb. ground beef
- One onion, chopped
- Two garlic cloves, minced
- 1 red bell pepper, chopped
- 1 green bell pepper, chopped
- 1 can (28 oz.) diced tomatoes, undrained
- 1 can (16 oz.) kidney beans, drained and rinsed
- 2 tbsp. chili powder
- 1 teaspoon. ground cumin
- 1 teaspoon. Paprika
- 1/2 teaspoon. Salt
- 1/4 teaspoon. black pepper

Instructions:

1. Cook the ground beef in a large saucepan over medium-high heat.

2. Add the onion, garlic, and red and green bell peppers to the saucepan and simmer until the veggies are soft.

3. Add the chopped tomatoes (with the liquid), kidney beans, chili powder, cumin, paprika, salt, and black pepper to the saucepan and mix thoroughly.

4. Bring the chili to a boil, then decrease the temperature to low and let it simmer for roughly 30 minutes.

2. Vegetarian Chili:

- One onion, chopped
- 1 green bell pepper, chopped
- 1 red bell pepper, chopped
- 2 garlic cloves, minced
- 2 cans (14 oz. each) diced tomatoes, undrained

- 2 cans (15 oz. each) kidney beans, drained and rinsed
- 1 can (15 oz.) black beans, drained and rinsed
- 1 can (15 oz.) corn, drained
- 2 tbsp. chili powder
- 1 tsp. ground cumin
- 1/2 tsp. paprika
- 1/2 tsp. salt
- 1/4 tsp. black pepper

Instructions:

1. Heat some oil in a big saucepan over medium heat.

2. Add the onion, green and red bell peppers, and garlic to the saucepan and simmer until the veggies are soft.

3. Add the chopped tomatoes (with the liquid), kidney beans, black beans, corn, chili powder, cumin, paprika, salt, and black pepper to the pot and combine completely.

4. Bring the chili to a boil, then decrease the temperature to low and let it simmer for roughly 30 minutes.

3. White Chicken Chili:

- One lb. boneless, skinless chicken breasts, cubed
- 1 onion, chopped
- 2 garlic cloves, minced
- 2 cans (15 oz. each) cannellini beans, strained and rinsed
- One can (4 oz) (4 oz.) of chopped green chilies
- One can (14 oz) (14 oz.) chicken broth
- 1 tsp. ground cumin
- 1/2 tsp. dried oregano
- 1/2 tsp. chili powder
- 1/4 tsp. Cayenne pepper \salt and black pepper to taste

Instructions:

1. Put some oil in a big saucepan over medium-high heat.
2. Add the chicken, onion, and garlic to the saucepan and simmer until the

chicken is browned and the onion is soft.

3. Add the cannellini beans, green chilies, chicken broth, cumin, oregano, chili powder, cayenne pepper, salt, and black pepper to the saucepan and mix thoroughly.

4. Bring the chili to a boil, then decrease the heat to low and let it boil for approximately 30 minutes.

5.0 PCOS-Friendly Dinner Recipes

5.1 Lean Protein-Based Recipes

Lean protein-based dishes are rich in protein yet low in fat and calories. They are perfect for anyone who wishes to gain muscle, shed weight, or maintain a balanced diet. These are some examples of lean protein-based recipes:

Grilled chicken breast with roasted veggies: Grilled chicken breast is a fantastic source of lean protein, while roasted vegetables are a tasty and healthful side dish. Season the chicken with salt, pepper, and herbs, and grill until cooked. Roast veggies such as broccoli, cauliflower, or carrots with little olive oil and spices until they are soft and caramelized.

Baked salmon with quinoa and vegetables: Salmon is another fantastic source of lean protein and healthy fats. Season the salmon with some lemon juice, garlic, and herbs, and bake it in the oven until it flakes easily with a fork. Serve it with quinoa, a great fiber and protein source, and steamed veggies such as asparagus or green beans.

Turkey and vegetable stir-fry: Ground turkey is a lean protein source that can be utilized in several cuisines. Prepare a stir-fry with turkey, bell peppers, onions, and mushrooms. Season it with ginger, garlic, and soy sauce, and serve it over brown rice or quinoa.

Grilled shrimp skewers with salad: Shrimp is a low-calorie and low-fat protein source of omega-3 fatty acids. Put some shrimp onto skewers, spray them with olive oil and pepper, then grill them until they are pink and cooked. Serve them with a side salad prepared with greens, veggies, and a light vinaigrette dressing.

Egg white omelet with vegetables: Egg whites are an excellent source of lean protein and are low in calories and fat. Prepare an omelet using egg whites and add veggies like spinach, tomatoes, and onions. Garnish it with some low-fat cheese or avocado for more taste and nutrients.

These lean protein-based meals are simple to create, tasty, and healthful. They are great for folks who wish to eat healthily and keep a balanced diet.

5.1.1 Grilled chicken breast with roasted veggies

Grilled chicken breast with roasted veggies is a healthy and easy-to-make dinner that is great for a lean protein-based diet. This is a dish that feeds four people:

Ingredients:

- Four boneless, skinless chicken breasts
- One red bell pepper, seeded and sliced
- One yellow bell pepper, seeded and sliced
- 1 red onion, sliced
- 2 zucchini, sliced
- 2 tablespoons olive oil
- Two cloves garlic, minced
- Salt and pepper to taste

Instructions:

1. Set the oven temperature to 425°F (218°C).

2. Whisk together the olive oil, garlic, salt, and pepper in a bowl.

3. Add the cut veggies to the bowl and toss to coat them evenly.

4. Arrange the veggies on a baking sheet in a single layer.

5. Bake the veggies for 20-25 minutes or until soft and gently browned.

6. When the veggies are cooking, fire up your grill over medium-high heat.

7. Garnish the chicken breasts with salt and pepper to taste.

8. Grill the chicken for 6-7 minutes on every side or until the internal temperature reaches 165°F (74°C).

9. After the chicken is done, let it rest for a few minutes before slicing it.

10. Serve the chicken with the roasted veggies on the side.

This meal is tasty and has an excellent dose of lean protein and fiber from roasted veggies. It's excellent for a healthy and fulfilling supper.

5.1.2 Baked salmon with quinoa and veggies

Here is a recipe for baked salmon with quinoa and vegetables:

Ingredients:

- 4 (4-6 ounce) salmon fillets
- 1 cup quinoa
- 2 cups water or chicken broth
- 2 cups chopped mixed veggies (such as bell peppers, zucchini, onion, and broccoli) (such as bell peppers, zucchini, onion, and broccoli)
- Two tablespoons of olive oil
- Salt and pepper to taste
- Lemon wedges for serving

Instructions:

1. Preheat oven to 375°F (190°C). Line a baking sheet with parchment paper.

2. Rinse the quinoa under cold water and add it to a saucepan with 2 cups of water or chicken stock. Bring to a boil, then decrease heat and simmer for 15-20 minutes or until thoroughly done.

3. Mix the chopped veggies in 1 tablespoon olive oil and season with salt and pepper.

4. Put the salmon fillets on the prepared baking sheet and season with salt and pepper. Sprinkle with leftover olive oil.

5. Place the seasoned veggies around the fish on the baking sheet.

6. Bake for 15-20 minutes until the fish is done and flakes readily with a fork.

7. Serve the salmon and veggies over a bed of quinoa. Sprinkle fresh lemon juice over the top of each serving.

This meal contains lean protein from the salmon and quinoa, while the mixed veggies add fiber and minerals.

5.1.3 Turkey and vegetable stir-fry

Here is a recipe for a nutritious and tasty turkey and veggie stir-fry:

Ingredients:

- 1 pound. ground turkey
- 2 cups mixed veggies (such as broccoli, carrots, snow peas, bell peppers, onions) (such as broccoli, carrots, snow peas, bell peppers onions)
- 1 tbsp. olive oil
- Two cloves garlic, minced
- 1 tbsp. ginger, minced
- 2 tbsp. low-sodium soy sauce
- 1 tbsp. honey
- 1 tsp. sesame oil
- Salt and pepper to taste

Instructions:

1. Heat olive oil in a large pan over medium-high heat.

2. Add ground turkey and sauté until browned, breaking it into little pieces as it cooks.

3. Once the turkey is cooked, add the mixed vegetables to the skillet and toss to integrate.

4. Add minced garlic and ginger to the pan and stir for 30 seconds until fragrant.

5. Mix soy sauce, honey, and sesame oil in a small bowl.

6. Pour the sauce over the turkey and vegetable mixture, and stir well to coat everything.

7. Cover the skillet and let everything cook for 5-7 minutes, or until the vegetables are tender and the turkey is fully cooked.

8. Serve the stir-fry over brown rice or quinoa, if desired.

This recipe is packed with lean protein from the ground turkey and plenty of nutritious veggies. The homemade stir-fry sauce adds a delicious and flavorful touch to the dish.

5.1.4 Grilled shrimp skewers with salad

Grilled shrimp skewers with salad is a tasty and healthful dinner that is great for any time of the year. Here is a recipe to help you prepare this dish:

Ingredients:

- One lb. big shrimp, peeled and deveined
- 1 tbsp. olive oil
- Two cloves garlic, minced
- 1 tsp. paprika
- 1/4 tsp. cayenne pepper
- Salt and black pepper to taste
- 2 cups mixed greens
- 1/2 red onion, sliced
- 1 avocado, sliced
- 1 pint cherry tomatoes, halved

- 1/4 cup chopped fresh cilantro
- 2 tbsp. lime juice
- 1 tbsp. honey
- 1 tbsp. olive oil

Instructions:

1. Preheat the grill to medium-high heat.

2. Whisk together olive oil, garlic, paprika, cayenne pepper, salt, and black pepper in a small bowl.

3. Thread shrimp on skewers and brush with the spice mixture.

4. Grill shrimp skewers on each side for 2-3 minutes until cooked through.

5. Mix mixed greens, red onion, avocado, cherry tomatoes, and cilantro in a large bowl.

6. Mix lime juice, honey, and olive oil in a separate bowl to create the dressing.

7. Pour the dressing over the salad and toss to coat.

8. Arrange the grilled shrimp skewers over the salad.

This dish is packed with protein and healthy fats, making it a fantastic alternative for a lean protein-based dinner. You may also add other veggies to the salad to improve the fiber and nutritious value of the meal. Enjoy!

5.2 Plant-Based Recipes

Plant-based recipes relate to meals oriented on plant-based items such as vegetables, fruits, grains, legumes, nuts, and seeds and may omit animal products or by-products such as meat, dairy, and eggs. Plant-based diets have been linked with several health advantages, including a lower risk of chronic illnesses such as heart disease, type 2 diabetes, and some forms of cancer.

These are some plant-based recipes:

Vegan Buddha Bowl: This is a colorful dish of veggies, grains, and plant-based protein. Start with a bed of cooked quinoa or brown rice and add roasted sweet potato, sautéed kale, sliced avocado, chickpeas, and a tahini dressing.

Lentil Curry: This rich and tasty meal may be served over rice or with naan bread. Boil lentils in a curry sauce prepared with coconut milk, tomato sauce, cumin, coriander, and turmeric. Throw in veggies such as carrots, spinach, and bell peppers for nourishment.

Chickpea Salad: This is a lovely and satisfying salad that can be served as a main meal or a side dish. Stir together canned chickpeas, chopped cucumber, diced tomato, sliced red onion, and a dressing prepared with olive oil, lemon juice, and dried herbs such as oregano or basil.

Tofu Stir-Fry: This is a fast and simple meal that may be modified with your favorite veggies. Sauté cubed tofu in a skillet with garlic, ginger, and soy sauce. Throw in veggies such as broccoli, bell peppers, and mushrooms, and serve over brown rice.

Vegan Chili: This is a substantial and tasty chili created using plant-based protein sources such as lentils or beans. Sauté the protein source with various veggies such as onion, bell peppers, and garlic, then throw in chopped tomatoes, tomato sauce, and a mixture of spices such as chili powder and cumin. Serve with avocado and cornbread for a full supper.

Here are a few plant-based meals that may be appreciated for their flavor and health advantages.

5.2.1 Vegan Buddha Bowl

Vegan Buddha Bowl is a colorful and healthy meal with various plant-based ingredients. Here is a recipe to make it:

Ingredients:

- 1 cup of quinoa
- One sweet potato, peeled and sliced
- 1 cup of broccoli florets
- 1 cup of sliced carrots
- 1 cup of sliced red cabbage

- One can of chickpeas, drained and rinsed
- One avocado, sliced
- 1/4 cup of tahini
- Two teaspoons of lemon juice
- Two teaspoons of water
- One tablespoon of olive oil
- Salt and pepper to taste

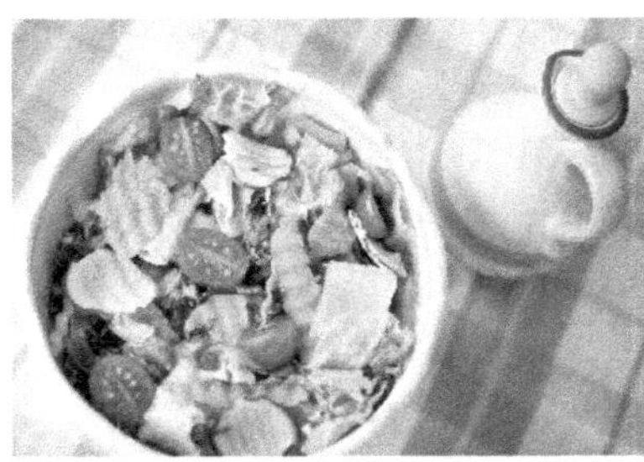

Instructions:

1. Cook quinoa according to the package directions.

2. Preheat the oven to 400°F.

3. Mix the sweet potato, broccoli, and carrots on a baking sheet with olive oil, salt, and pepper. Roast for 20-25 minutes or until tender.

4. Combine tahini, lemon juice, water, salt, and pepper in a separate bowl to create the dressing.

5. To create the dish, split quinoa among four bowls, then top it with

roasted veggies, chickpeas, red cabbage, and avocado. Drizzle with tahini dressing.

Enjoy your tasty and nutritious Vegan Buddha Bowl!

5.2.2 Lentil Curry

Lentil curry is a tasty and nutritious plant-based recipe that is excellent for a healthy evening. Here's a recipe for lentil curry:

Ingredients:

- 1 cup dried brown or green lentils, washed
- One tablespoon of olive oil
- One onion, chopped
- Three cloves garlic, minced
- One tablespoon of curry powder
- One teaspoon of ground cumin
- 1/2 teaspoon ground turmeric
- 1/4 teaspoon ground cinnamon
- 1/4 teaspoon ground cloves
- One can (14.5 ounces) of chopped tomatoes, undrained
- One can (13.5 ounces) of coconut milk

- 2 cups vegetable broth
- Salt and black pepper, to taste
- Fresh cilantro, chopped, for garnish (optional)

Instructions:

1. In a large saucepan, heat the olive oil over medium heat. Add the onion, garlic, and sauté until soft and aromatic for approximately 5 minutes.

2. Add the curry powder, cumin, turmeric, cinnamon, and cloves and simmer, frequently stirring, for 1 minute.

3. Add the lentils, chopped tomatoes (with their liquid), coconut milk, and vegetable broth. Stir to mix.

4. Bring the mixture to a boil, then decrease the heat to low and simmer, covered, until the lentils are cooked, and the curry has thickened, approximately 30 minutes.

5. Season with salt and black pepper to taste. Serve hot, garnished with chopped cilantro if desired.

This lentil curry is rich in plant-based protein and fiber from the lentils, and the spices give a ton of flavor and antioxidants. It's also gluten-free and vegan, so it's a wonderful alternative for anyone with dietary limitations. Serve it with brown rice or some naan bread for a full and fulfilling supper.

5.2.3 Chickpea Salad

Chickpea salad is a tasty and healthful plant-based meal that is simple to cook and excellent for lunch or supper. It's also a terrific meal for potlucks or picnics since it's simple to carry and can be served cold or at room temperature.

To prepare a chickpea salad, drain and wash a can of chickpeas. Next, cut up some fresh veggies such as cucumber, tomato, and red onion. For added taste, you may also add some chopped fresh herbs like parsley or cilantro.

Then, whisk up a simple dressing of olive oil, lemon juice, and a touch of salt and pepper. Toss the chickpeas and veggies in the dressing until everything is completely covered.

To give some more texture and taste, you may also put in some chopped nuts or seeds like almonds or sunflower seeds. Add some crumbled feta cheese or sliced avocado for extra richness.

After everything is incorporated, let the salad cool in the fridge for at least 30 minutes to let the flavors melt together. Serve the chickpea salad chilled or at room temperature, and enjoy!

Here's an example recipe for chickpea salad:

Ingredients:

- One can of chickpeas, drained and rinsed
- 1 small cucumber, diced \s1 big tomato, diced
- 1/4 red onion, diced
- 1/4 cup chopped fresh parsley
- 1/4 cup chopped almonds
- 2 tbsp olive oil
- 1 tbsp lemon juice
- Salt & pepper, to taste

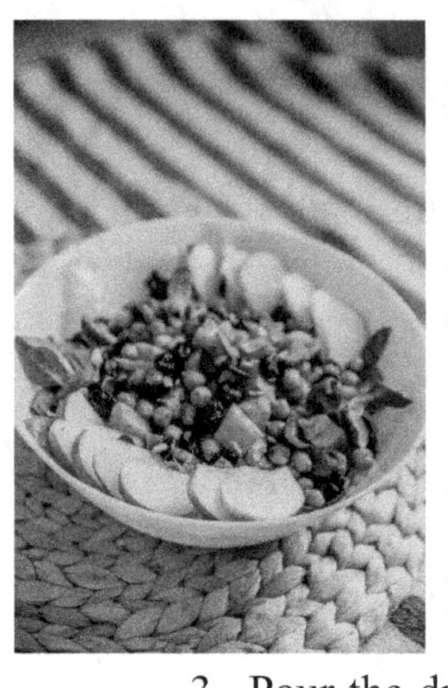

Directions:

1. Mix chickpeas, cucumber, tomato, red onion, and parsley in a large bowl.

2. Mix the olive oil, lemon juice, salt, and pepper in a small bowl.

3. Pour the dressing over the chickpea mixture and toss to coat.

4. Add the chopped almonds and mix again.

5. Cover the bowl with plastic wrap and chill for at least 30 minutes.

6. Serve the chickpea salad chilled or at room temperature.

Vegan chili is a substantial and healthy dinner for chilly winter days. This dish is perfect for individuals who follow a plant-based diet since it lacks animal ingredients. Here's a recipe for vegan chili with a storyline:

Ingredients:

- Two tablespoons of olive oil
- 1 onion, chopped
- 3 garlic cloves, minced
- 1 red bell pepper, chopped
- 1 green bell pepper, chopped
- 1 jalapeño pepper, chopped
- 2 teaspoons chili powder
- Two tablespoons of ground cumin
- One teaspoon of smoked paprika
- 1/2 teaspoon cayenne pepper
- Two cans (15 ounces each) of black beans, drained and rinsed
- Two cans (15 ounces each) of kidney beans, drained and rinsed
- One can (28 ounces) (28 ounces) smashed tomatoes
- 1 cup water

- Salt and pepper to taste

Instructions:

1. Heat the olive oil in a big saucepan over medium heat. Add the onion and garlic, and sauté for 3-4 minutes, or until the onion is transparent.

2. Add the red bell pepper, green bell pepper, and jalapeño pepper to the saucepan. Sauté for another 5-7 minutes or until the peppers are soft.

3. Add the chili powder, ground cumin, smoked paprika, and cayenne pepper to the saucepan. Stir until the veggies are covered with the seasonings.

4. Add the black beans, kidney beans, crushed tomatoes, and water to the pot. Stir until everything is completely blended.

5. Bring the chili to a boil, then decrease the heat to low. Cook for 30-40 minutes, stirring regularly, or

until the chili has thickened to your desired consistency.

6. Season the chili with salt and pepper to taste.

7. Serve the chili hot, topped with vegan sour cream, chopped cilantro, and sliced avocado.

Growing up, chili was a regular dinner in my home. My mother used to cook a hearty beef chili full of rich flavors and spices. Nevertheless, when I embraced a vegan diet, I had to find a new way to enjoy this favorite meal. That's when I came into this vegan chili recipe. It's full of protein-rich beans, nutrient-dense veggies, and a wonderful combination of spices. Moreover, it's really simple to make! Every time I eat this chili, it reminds me of my childhood's warmth and comfort while giving me the nutrients I need to flourish on a plant-based diet.

One-pot dinners are recipes made in a single pot or skillet, making them a quick and practical alternative for hectic weeknights. They often include integrating protein, veggies, and carbohydrates into one meal, which means less cleaning and fewer dishes to wash. These are some examples of one-pot meals:

Chicken and Rice: In a large saucepan or Dutch oven, sauté chopped onions and garlic until aromatic. Add chicken pieces and brown on both sides. Add diced tomatoes, chicken broth, and uncooked rice. Bring to a boil, then decrease the heat to low and cover. Simmer for approximately 20 minutes or until the rice is soft and the chicken is cooked.

Beef Stroganoff: Brown sliced meat in a large pan. Add sliced mushrooms and chopped onions and sauté until soft. Mix in beef broth, sour cream, and egg noodles. Bring to a boil, then decrease heat and simmer until the noodles are done, and the sauce has thickened.

Vegetable Soup: In a large pot or Dutch oven, sauté chopped onions and garlic until aromatic. Add chopped veggies, such as carrots, celery, and potatoes. Pour in veggie broth and add canned chopped tomatoes. Bring to a boil, decrease heat, and simmer until the veggies are soft.

Shakshuka: In a large pan, sauté chopped onions and bell peppers until soft. Add canned diced tomatoes, cumin, paprika, and cayenne pepper. Break eggs immediately into the skillet, cover, and cook until the whites are set, and the yolks are still runny. Serve with fresh bread for dipping.

Jambalaya: In a large pot or Dutch oven, sauté chopped onions, bell peppers, and celery until soft. Add diced chicken and sliced smoked sausage and heat until browned. Add diced tomatoes, chicken broth, and uncooked rice. Bring to a boil, then decrease the heat to low and cover. Simmer for approximately 20 minutes or until the rice is soft and the chicken is cooked.

These one-pot dinners may be adjusted with various meats, veggies, and spices to fit your taste preferences. They are also perfect for meal prep and leftovers since they can be readily reheated for a fast, nutritious lunch or supper.

6.0 PCOS-Friendly Snack Recipes

6.1 Nutrient-Dense Snack Ideas

Nutrient-dense snack choices are a terrific way to feed your body with critical vitamins and minerals throughout the day. Here are several examples:

Hard-boiled eggs: Eggs are a terrific source of protein, healthy fats, and various vitamins and minerals, making them an ideal nutrient-dense snack.

Mixed nuts: A combination of almonds, walnuts, pistachios, cashews, and peanuts may supply your body with a nice dosage of healthy fats, protein, fiber, and numerous vitamins and minerals.

Greek yogurt with berries: Greek yogurt is strong in protein and low in sugar, and when mixed with antioxidant-rich berries, it makes for a fantastic nutrient-dense snack.

Hummus with veggies: Hummus is a tasty and nutrient-dense dip that may be coupled with sliced carrots, cucumbers, bell peppers, and other vegetables for a nutritious snack.

Apple slices with almond butter: Apples are strong in fiber, while almond butter delivers protein, healthy fats, and critical minerals.

Edamame: Edamame is a low-calorie, high-protein snack rich in fiber, vitamins, and minerals.

Roasted chickpeas: Roasted chickpeas are crispy, delicious, and full of fiber, protein, and other key elements.

Cottage cheese with fruit: Cottage cheese is a low-fat, high-protein snack with fresh fruit, such as berries or sliced peaches.

Kale chips: Kale is a nutritious powerhouse, and when roasted in the oven with a little olive oil, it produces a crispy and tasty snack.

Dark chocolate: Dark chocolate includes antioxidants and is a rich source of iron, magnesium, and zinc, making it a fantastic nutrient-dense treat in moderation.

Here are a few examples of nutrient-dense snack options that may give your body critical vitamins and minerals throughout the day.

6.2 Low-Carb Snack Ideas

Low-carb snacks are a terrific method to satisfy hunger and maintain energy levels between meals while supporting a low-carb diet. Here are some options for low-carb snacks:

Nuts and seeds: They are strong in healthy fats, protein, and fiber, making them a terrific snack option. Almonds, walnuts, pecans, pistachios, pumpkin seeds, and sunflower seeds are all low in carbohydrates and may be consumed raw or roasted.

Vegetables and dip: Vegetables are low in carbohydrates and rich in fiber and other nutrients. Eat them raw or mildly steamed with a dip prepared from sour cream, hummus, guacamole, or salsa.

Hard-boiled eggs: Hard-boiled eggs are a handy and pleasant snack. They are strong in protein and healthy fats and may be seasoned with salt, pepper, or other spices.

Cheese and meat: Cheese and meat are fantastic protein sources and healthy fats. Eat pieces of cheese with salami, pepperoni, or deli meat.

Avocado: Avocado is an excellent source of healthy fats and fiber. Eat it sliced with salt & pepper or mixed into guacamole.

Greek yogurt: Greek yogurt is strong in protein and low in carbohydrates. Eat it simply or with a few berries for additional taste.

Edamame: Edamame is a wonderful source of protein and fiber. Boil or steam the pods and eat them as a snack.

Low-carb protein bars: Several low-carb protein bars available on the market may be a practical and fulfilling snack.

Remember, while picking low-carb snacks, choosing whole, minimally processed foods and controlling portion sizes is crucial to keep inside your daily carb allowance.

6.2.1 Nuts and seeds

Nuts and seeds are excellent sources of nutrients and healthy fats. They are a terrific supplement to a healthy diet and may be utilized in several ways. Here are several examples:

Almonds: Almonds are a fantastic source of vitamin E and healthy fats. They may be consumed as a snack, added to smoothies, or used to create almond butter.

Walnuts: Walnuts are abundant in omega-3 fatty acids and antioxidants. They may be added to salads and porridge or used to create walnut pesto.

Chia seeds: Chia seeds are a rich source of fiber, protein, and omega-3 fatty acids. They may be added to smoothies and yogurt or used to create chia pudding.

Flax seeds are rich in fiber, omega-3 fatty acids, and lignans. They may be added to smoothies and porridge or used to create flaxseed crackers.

Pumpkin seeds: Pumpkin seeds are abundant in magnesium, zinc, and protein. They may be roasted and eaten as a snack or added to salads.

Sunflower seeds: Sunflower seeds are rich in vitamin E and selenium. They may be consumed as a snack, added to trail mix, or used to create sunflower seed butter.

Overall, nuts and seeds are a terrific supplement to a healthy diet and may be utilized in a number of ways to add taste, texture, and nutrients to meals and snacks.

6.3 Sweet and Savory Snack Recipes

Here are some examples of sweet and savory snack recipes:

Sweet Potato Toast with Avocado and Egg:

- Slice a sweet potato into 1/4-inch-thick slices.

- Toast them in the oven or toaster.
- Top with mashed avocado and a fried or poached egg.

Baked Sweet Potato Chips: Thinly slice a sweet potato, mix it with olive oil and salt, and bake in the oven until crispy.

Apple Chips with Cinnamon: Slice apples thinly, sprinkle with cinnamon, and bake in the oven until crispy.

Ants on a Log: Put almond butter on celery sticks and sprinkle with raisins or dried cranberries.

Roasted Chickpeas: Mix chickpeas with olive oil and spices, such as cumin or smoky paprika, and bake in the oven until crispy.

Caprese Skewers: Thread cherry tomatoes, fresh mozzarella, and basil leaves onto skewers and sprinkle with balsamic sauce.

Trail Mix: Blend nuts, seeds, dried fruit, and dark chocolate chips for a protein-packed and enjoyable snack.

Cheese and Apple Slices: Combine apple slices with your favorite cheese for a sweet and delicious snack.

Avocado & Tomato Toast:

- Toast a piece of bread.
- Put mashed avocado on top.
- Add sliced tomatoes and a sprinkling of salt and pepper.

Savory Greek Yogurt Dip: Combine Greek yogurt with chopped herbs, such as dill or chives, and serve with sliced vegetables or whole-grain crackers for dipping.

These snacks contain protein, fiber, and healthy fats to keep you full and satisfied between meals.

6.3.1 Cooked Sweet Potato Chips:

Baked Sweet Potato Chips are a tasty and healthful alternative to typical potato chips. They are simple to prepare and may be eaten as a snack or side dish. Here is a recipe for Baked Sweet Potato Chips with a storyline:

Ingredients:

- Two medium-sized sweet potatoes
- Two tablespoons of olive oil
- 1 teaspoon salt \s1/2 teaspoon black pepper
- 1/2 teaspoon paprika
- 1/4 teaspoon garlic powder

Instructions:

1. Preheat your oven to 375°F (190°C).

2. Peel the sweet potatoes and slice them into thin, even rounds using a sharp knife or a mandolin slicer.

3. Whisk together the olive oil, salt, pepper, paprika, and garlic powder in a small bowl.

4. Put the sweet potato slices in a big basin and pour the seasoned oil mixture over them. Toss to coat the slices evenly.

5. Place the sweet potato slices in a single layer on a baking sheet coated with parchment paper.

6. Bake the sweet potato chips in the oven for 20-25 minutes or until they are crispy and golden brown.

7. Remove the baking sheet from the oven and let the sweet potato chips cool for a few minutes before serving.

Sophie was always looking for healthy snack options that she could enjoy guilt-free. One day, while perusing through a cooking magazine, she came onto a Baked Sweet Potato Chips recipe. Impressed by the concept, she decided to try making them at home. When she cut the sweet potatoes into thin rounds, the brilliant orange color of the vegetable attracted her eye, making her even more enthusiastic about sampling the chips.

As they were seasoned and baked, the spices filled her kitchen, wetting her mouth. When she took her first mouthful, she was pleased by the crunchiness of the chips and the delightful blend of sweet and salty tastes. Sophie felt happy for herself for attempting something new and producing a nutritious snack she could enjoy anytime.

Ants on a Log is a popular snack prepared by filling celery sticks with nut butter (such as peanut butter or almond butter) and topping them with raisins or other tiny dried fruit to mimic "ants." Here's a basic recipe:

Ingredients:

- Celery sticks
- Nut butter of your choosing (peanut butter, almond butter, cashew butter, etc.) (peanut butter, almond butter, cashew butter, etc.)
- Raisins or other tiny dried fruit

Instructions:

1. Wash and dry the celery sticks.

2. Cut the celery sticks into 3-4 inch pieces.

3. Put a layer of nut butter into the celery sticks, filling the empty middle.

4. Put raisins or other tiny dried fruit on top of the nut butter, pushing them in slightly to help them stay.

5. Repeat with the remaining celery sticks and serve.

This snack is tasty and nutritional, delivering a wonderful combination of fiber, healthy fats, and protein. It's a terrific alternative for kids and adults alike and can be easily adjusted to suit your preferences by adding other kinds of nut butter or dried fruit.

6.3.3 Roasted Chickpeas

Roasted chickpeas are a nutritious and pleasant snack that can be cooked quickly at home. Here's a basic recipe:

Ingredients:

- One can of chickpeas (15 oz) (15 oz.)
- One tablespoon of olive oil
- Salt and pepper to taste

- Optional seasonings: garlic powder, cumin, paprika, chili powder, or any additional spice of your choosing

Instructions:

1. Preheat the oven to 400°F (200°C).

2. Rinse and drain the chickpeas, then pat them dry with a paper towel.

3. Put the chickpeas in a mixing bowl, then add the olive oil, salt, pepper, and other ingredients.

4. Stir the chickpeas until they are uniformly covered with the spice mixture.

5. Spread the chickpeas out in a single layer on a baking sheet.

6. Roast the chickpeas in the oven for 20-30 minutes or until they are crispy and golden brown.

7. Take the chickpeas from the oven and allow them to cool for a few minutes before serving.

Roasted chickpeas are a flexible snack that may be modified to your liking. You may experiment with various spices to produce sweet or savory tastes. For example, you may add cinnamon and sugar for a sweet snack or curry powder for a savory one. Enjoy!

6.3.4 Caprese Skewers

Caprese skewers are a simple and tasty snack that is excellent for summer entertaining or as a light starter. Here's a recipe for Caprese skewers:

Ingredients:

- Cherry tomatoes
- Fresh basil leaves
- Fresh mozzarella balls
- Balsamic glaze
- Skewers

Instructions:

1. Start by cleaning the cherry tomatoes and basil leaves.

2. Cut the mozzarella balls into bite-sized pieces.

3. Thread one cherry tomato, one slice of mozzarella, and one basil leaf onto each skewer.

4. Drizzle the skewers with balsamic glaze shortly before serving.

5. Serve and enjoy!

Caprese skewers blend luscious cherry tomatoes, creamy mozzarella, and aromatic basil; all finished with a sweet and tangy balsamic sauce. These are crowd-pleasing snack that is guaranteed to wow!

6.3.5 Avocado with Tomato Toast

Avocado and Tomato Toast is a tasty and healthy snack or light supper that is simple to make and suitable for any time of day. The combination of creamy avocado and juicy tomato is traditional, and when coupled with a piece of substantial bread, it makes for a pleasant and savory snack.

To prepare Avocado and Tomato Toast, you will need the following ingredients:

- One ripe avocado
- One big tomato
- Two pieces of whole-grain bread
- Salt & pepper, to taste
- Optional toppings: sliced red onion, crumbled feta cheese, chopped fresh cilantro

Instructions:

1. Preheat the oven to 400 degrees F (200 degrees C) (200 degrees C).

2. Split the avocado in half and remove the pit. Scrape the meat into a small dish and mash it with a fork until smooth.

3. Chop the tomato into thin pieces.

4. Toast the bread until it is crispy and golden brown.

5. Put the mashed avocado onto each piece of bread.

6. Put the tomato slices on top of the avocado, overlapping them slightly.

7. Season with salt and pepper, to taste.

8. If preferred, sprinkle with extra toppings, such as sliced red onion, crumbled feta cheese, or chopped fresh cilantro.

9. Serve immediately and enjoy!

Sophie was seeking a fast and simple snack to enjoy between meals. She had a ripe avocado and some fresh tomatoes, so she prepared Avocado and Tomato Toast. Sophie warmed the oven and split the avocado in half, removing the pit and putting the flesh into a basin. She mashed the avocado with a fork until it was smooth and chopped the tomato into thin slices.

Then, Sophie toasted two pieces of whole-grain bread until they were crispy and golden brown. She poured the mashed avocado over each piece of bread and positioned the tomato slices on top, overlapping them slightly. Sophie seasoned the bread with salt and pepper, then added some sliced red onion, crumbled feta cheese, and chopped fresh cilantro for more flavor and texture.

Sophie tasted her Avocado & Tomato Toast and was instantly thrilled with the blend of flavors and textures. The creamy avocado, juicy tomato, and crunchy toast combined for a fulfilling, delightful snack filled with nutrients. She kept the second piece for later and felt comfortable knowing she had a healthy and delicious snack alternative whenever hunger arose.

7.0 PCOS-Friendly Dessert Recipes

7.1 Low-Sugar Dessert Choices

Low-sugar desserts are a terrific way to satisfy your sweet taste without ingesting excessive quantities of sugar. Here are some possibilities for low-sugar desserts:

Fresh Fruit Salad: Fresh fruit is inherently delicious and includes natural sugars, fiber, and antioxidants. Mix a range of bright fruits such as berries, sliced kiwi, and mangoes for a delightful and healthful dessert.

Greek Yogurt with Berries: Greek yogurt is an excellent protein source and low in sugar. Top it up with fresh berries like blueberries, raspberries, or strawberries to add natural sweetness.

Chocolate Chia Pudding: Mix chia seeds, almond milk, unsweetened cocoa powder, and a sugar replacement to produce a chocolaty, protein-packed pudding low in sugar.

Baked Apples: Slice apples and sprinkle them with cinnamon, then bake them in the oven until soft. This low-sugar dessert is pleasant and may be served hot or cold.

No-Bake Energy Balls - Mix dates, nuts, and your favorite mix-ins like coconut flakes, cocoa powder, or almond butter, and make them into balls. These energy balls are great for appeasing your sweet craving and offering a surge of energy.

Banana Lovely Cream: Peel and freeze ripe bananas, then combine them in a food processor until smooth and creamy. This low-sugar delicacy has a texture comparable to ice cream but is significantly healthier.

Peanut Butter Cookies: Mix peanut butter, almond flour, and a sugar replacement to produce low-sugar, high-protein cookies that are both tasty and gratifying.

Berry Sorbet - Mix frozen berries with a sugar substitute and a small amount of water until smooth. This low-sugar dish is a delicious and healthful alternative to regular sorbet.

Dark Chocolate Bark: Melt dark chocolate and stir with your preferred nuts and dried fruits, then spread the mixture onto a parchment-lined baking sheet and freeze until hard. This low-sugar dessert is excellent for satisfying your appetite and offering antioxidants and healthy fats.

Cinnamon Baked Pears: Slice and sprinkle them with cinnamon, then bake in the oven until soft. This low-sugar dessert is warm and soothing and may be served with whipped cream or yogurt.

7.1.1 Fresh Fruit Salad

Fresh fruit salad is a nutritious and pleasant treat that can be eaten any time of the year. It's a terrific way to enjoy a variety of fruits and receive a decent dose of vitamins and fiber. Here's an easy recipe for a fresh fruit salad:

Ingredients:

- 2 cups of chopped fresh fruit (such as strawberries, blueberries, kiwi, pineapple, mango, and grapes) (such as strawberries, blueberries, kiwi, pineapple, mango, and grapes)

- 1 spoonful of honey

- One tablespoon of fresh lime juice

- 1/4 cup of fresh mint leaves, chopped (optional) (optional)

Instructions:

1. Wash and cut the fruit into bite-sized pieces.

2. Mix the honey and lime juice in a separate bowl to create the dressing.

3. Mix the fruit and dressing in a large bowl and gently toss until the fruit is covered with the dressing.

4. Garnish with chopped mint leaves (optional) (optional).

Mary was having a summer BBQ party and wanted to provide a nutritious and refreshing dessert that everyone would appreciate. She decided to prepare a fresh fruit salad, using a variety of fruits that were in season. She went to the local farmers market and picked up some fresh strawberries, blueberries, kiwi, pineapple, mango, and grapes.

When Mary returned home, she cleaned and sliced the fruit into bite-sized pieces. She produced a simple dressing by mixing honey and lime juice. She then put the fruit and dressing in a big dish, gently tossing everything together until the dressing covered the fruit. Mary also opted to add some chopped mint leaves for a fresh and tasty accent.

The fresh fruit salad was a smash at the celebration, and everyone appreciated the range of sweet and tart tastes. Mary was glad to give a nutritious, tasty dessert that was great for the summer heat. She even had some leftovers, which she loved for breakfast the following day.

Greek Yogurt with Berries is a nutritious and tasty snack that may fulfill your sweet taste while giving various health advantages. Here is a recipe with a step-by-step tutorial on how to prepare this easy but wonderful snack:

Ingredients:

- 1 cup of Greek yogurt
- 1 cup of mixed berries (such as strawberries, blueberries, raspberries, and blackberries) (such as strawberries, blueberries, raspberries, and blackberries)
- 1-2 teaspoons of honey (optional) (optional)

Instructions:

1. Rinse the mixed berries under cold water and blot them dry with a paper towel.

2. Chop the strawberries into tiny pieces.

3. Mix the Greek yogurt and honey (if using) in a mixing bowl until thoroughly blended.

4. Add the mixed berries to the yogurt mixture and stir gently until the berries are uniformly distributed.

5. Serve the yogurt and fruit combination in a dish or cup.

You may also adapt this recipe by adding extra toppings like granola, nuts, or seeds. This snack is a fantastic source of protein, calcium, and antioxidants, making it a nutritious and tasty alternative for any time of the day.

7.1.3 Chocolate Chia Pudding

Chocolate chia pudding is a tasty and nutritious dessert option that is simple to create and filled with nutrients. Here's a recipe for creating chocolate chia pudding:

Ingredients:

- 1/4 cup chia seeds
- 1 cup unsweetened almond milk
- One tablespoon of cocoa powder
- One tablespoon of maple syrup or honey
- 1/2 teaspoon vanilla extract

- Pinch of salt

Instructions:

1. In a dish, stir together chia seeds, almond milk, chocolate powder, maple syrup or honey, vanilla extract, and salt until completely incorporated.

2. Cover the bowl and refrigerate for at least 2 hours or overnight, stirring regularly.

3. After the pudding has thickened and the chia seeds have absorbed the liquid, please thoroughly toss it to break up any clumps.

4. If preferred, serve the pudding topped with fresh fruit, nuts, or coconut flakes.

You may also experiment with other tastes by adding ingredients like cinnamon, nut butter, or espresso powder to the batter. Enjoy your chocolate chia pudding as a healthy and enjoyable dessert or snack!

Baked apples are a tasty and easy-to-make dessert that is excellent for any occasion. They may be produced with only a few basic ingredients and are a healthier alternative to regular baked items. Here's a recipe for baked apples:

Ingredients:

- Four medium-sized apples
- 1/4 cup brown sugar
- 1/4 cup rolled oats
- 1/4 cup chopped nuts (pecans or walnuts work nicely) (pecans or walnuts work well)
- 1/2 teaspoon cinnamon
- 1/4 teaspoon nutmeg
- Two teaspoons of melted butter
- 1/2 cup water

Instructions:

1. Preheat the oven to 375°F.

2. Core the apples and arrange them in a baking dish.

3. Mix the brown sugar, rolled oats, chopped almonds, cinnamon, nutmeg, and melted butter in a small bowl.

4. Put the mixture into the middle of each apple.

5. Pour the water into the bottom of the baking dish.

6. Cover the dish with aluminum foil and bake for 25-30 minutes.

7. Remove the foil and bake for 10-15 minutes, until the apples are soft and the topping is golden brown.

8. Serve the baked apples warm, with a scoop of vanilla ice cream or a dollop of whipped cream, if preferred.

Baked apples are a terrific way to enjoy a delicious treat without ingesting too much sugar or bad fats. These are also flexible treats since you can personalize the filling with your favorite ingredients, such as raisins, dried cranberries, or sliced dates. Also, you may use other types of apples, such as Honeycrisp, Granny Smith, or

Gala, to provide a distinct taste and texture to the meal.

Cinnamon Baked Pears are an easy and tasty low-sugar dessert alternative. This dish uses luscious pears and toasty cinnamon spices for a soothing and healthful dessert.

Ingredients:

- Four ripe pears
- One tablespoon of melted coconut oil
- One teaspoon of ground cinnamon
- 1/4 teaspoon ground nutmeg
- One tablespoon honey or maple syrup (optional)
- Chopped nuts or granola for topping (optional)
-

Instructions:

1. Preheat the oven to 375°F.

2. Split the pears in half lengthwise and remove the core and seeds with a spoon.

3. Put the pears cut side up on a baking dish or a baking sheet coated with parchment paper.

4. Pour the melted coconut oil over the pears, then sprinkle the cinnamon and nutmeg.

5. If preferred, sprinkle honey or maple syrup over the top of the pears for extra sweetness.

6. Bake the pears for 20-25 minutes or until soft and gently browned.

7. Serve the pears warm, topped with chopped nuts or granola if preferred.

Growing up, my grandma cooked the most incredible cinnamon-baked pears for dessert. As a youngster, I was always astounded at how such a simple and healthful dessert could be so wonderful.

As an adult, I cook this dish for myself and my family. It's a fantastic dessert alternative for individuals who want something sweet and comforting without all the extra sugar and calories of typical sweets. The warm cinnamon flavor blends nicely with the natural sweetness of the pears, making this meal a favorite for all seasons.

Fruit-based desserts are a terrific way to satisfy your sweet taste while adding nutritional components. These are some recipes for fruit-based desserts:

Berry Parfait: Combine mixed berries, Greek yogurt, and granola in a glass or container for a nutritious and tasty parfait.

Grilled Pineapple: Cut pineapple into pieces and grill until caramelized. Serve with a dollop of whipped cream or coconut cream and a sprinkling of cinnamon.

Fruit Skewers: Thread strawberries, pineapple, and kiwi onto skewers for a colorful and healthful dessert. You may also sprinkle it with honey or melted dark chocolate.

Mixed Berry Crisp: Blend mixed berries with sugar, lemon juice, and cornstarch. Cover with oats, flour, butter, and brown sugar, and bake until golden brown.

Mango Coconut Chia Pudding:
1. Mix chia seeds, coconut milk, and honey in a bowl.
2. Add chopped mango and stir.
3. Let the mixture lie for a few hours or overnight in the fridge until the chia seeds have absorbed the liquid and the pudding has thickened.

Fruit Salad with Honey-Lime Dressing: Mix your favorite fruits, such as watermelon, cantaloupe, kiwi, and berries. Drizzle with a dressing prepared from honey, lime juice, and mint.

Grilled Peaches with Honey and Yogurt: Cut peaches in half and grill until soft. Serve with a dollop of Greek yogurt, a honey drizzle, and chopped nuts sprinkling.

Frozen Yogurt Bark:
1. Combine Greek yogurt, honey, and favorite fruits like blueberries and strawberries.

2. Spread the mixture onto a baking sheet and freeze until firm.
3. Cut into pieces and serve as a nutritious and refreshing dessert.

Banana Ice Cream: Mix frozen bananas in a food processor until creamy and smooth. You may also add chocolate powder or peanut butter for extra taste.

Baked Apples: Core apples and fill with a combination of oats, cinnamon, and chopped almonds. Bake until soft and serve with a whipped or vanilla ice cream dab.

These fruit-based treats are tasty and rich in minerals and vitamins.

7.2.1 Berry Parfait

Berry parfait is a tasty and healthy dessert that is suitable for any occasion. It is a layered dessert that mixes fresh berries, yogurt, and granola, making it a nutritious and delightful treat.

Here's an easy recipe for a berry parfait:

Ingredients:

- 1 cup fresh berries (strawberries, blueberries, raspberries, or any other berries of your choosing) (strawberries, blueberries, raspberries, or any other berries of your choice)
- 1 cup plain Greek yogurt
- 1/2 cup granola
- One tablespoon honey (optional) (optional)

Instructions:

1. Wash and slice the berries into tiny pieces.

2. In a small dish, combine the Greek yogurt with honey (if using) (if using).

3. In a large glass or jar, start stacking the ingredients. Begin with a layer of yogurt, a layer of berries, and then a layer of granola. Continue until you reach the top of the glass, being sure to conclude with a layer of granola.

4. Serve immediately or cover and chill until ready to serve.

You can also customize this recipe by adding different fruits, using flavored yogurt, or swapping out the granola for other toppings like nuts or coconut flakes. Enjoy!

7.2.2 Mixed Berry Crisp

Mixed berry crisp is a tasty delicacy that is great for berry season. It's a simple dish that may be created with various berries, such as blueberries, raspberries, strawberries, and blackberries. The crisp is constructed with a buttery coating and a delicious berry filling.

Here's a recipe for mixed berry crisp:

Ingredients:

- 6 cups mixed berries
- 1/3 cup sugar
- 1 tbsp cornstarch
- 1/2 tsp vanilla extract
- 1/2 cup flour
- 1/2 cup rolled oats
- 1/2 cup brown sugar
- 1/2 tsp cinnamon

- 1/4 tsp salt
- 1/2 cup unsalted butter, sliced into tiny pieces

Instructions:

1. Preheat oven to 375°F.

2. Whisk together the berries, sugar, cornstarch, and vanilla essence in a dish. Spoon the mixture into a 9-inch baking dish.

3. Whisk together the flour, rolled oats, brown sugar, cinnamon, and salt in another dish. Add the butter and use your hands to stir until the mixture is crumbly.

4. Sprinkle the crumbly mixture over the top of the berry mixture.

5. Bake for 30-40 minutes, until the top, is golden brown and the berry filling is bubbling.

6. Let the crisp cool for a few minutes before serving it with whipped cream or vanilla ice cream.

Enjoy your wonderful mixed berry crisp!

7.2.3 Mango Coconut Chia Pudding

Mango Coconut Chia Pudding is a tasty and healthful dish that is excellent for anybody who enjoys tropical tastes. It's created with chia seeds, which are full of fiber and protein, and coconut milk, which lends a rich and creamy texture. The addition of fresh mango gives it a blast of sweetness and tropical taste.

Ingredients:

- 1/2 cup chia seeds
- 2 cups coconut milk
- 1/4 cup honey or maple syrup
- 1 tsp vanilla extract
- 1 big ripe mango, peeled and chopped
- Unsweetened shredded coconut, for topping

Instructions:

1. In a large mixing bowl, whisk together the chia seeds, coconut milk, honey or maple syrup, and vanilla extract until well

combined. Cover the bowl with plastic wrap and refrigerate for at least 2 hours or overnight.

2. After the chia pudding has been set, please give it a thorough swirl to ensure it's uniformly blended. If the pudding is too thick, add more coconut milk to thin it down.

3. Divide the chia pudding into four dishes or jars to construct the pudding. Garnish each dish with a big scoop of diced mango and a sprinkling of unsweetened shredded coconut.

4. Serve the mango coconut chia pudding immediately, or preserve it in the refrigerator for up to 3 days.

Mango Coconut Chia Pudding is a fantastic nutritious, refreshing dessert you can enjoy any time of day. It's particularly nice when you're yearning for something sweet and tropical during hot summer days. You may even prep it the night before and consume it for breakfast or as a lunchtime snack. The mix of chia seeds, coconut milk, and fresh mango is a wonderful balance of texture and taste. Additionally, it's vegan and gluten-free, making it a treat everyone can enjoy.

7.2.4 Banana Ice Cream

Banana ice cream is a healthy and tasty alternative to classic ice cream. It is produced with frozen bananas that are pureed till smooth and creamy. The outcome is a delicious and delightful dessert with minimal calories and fat.

To create banana ice cream, start by peeling ripe bananas and chopping them into tiny pieces. Put the banana slices in a resealable plastic bag and freeze for at least 2 hours or overnight. After freezing the bananas, please put them in a blender or food processor and puree until smooth and creamy. You may need to pause and scrape down the sides of the blender or food processor to ensure all the pieces are pureed.

There are various versions you may try with banana ice cream, such as:

Chocolate banana ice cream: Add a spoonful of cocoa powder or chocolate chips to the blender before mixing for a chocolate taste.

Peanut butter banana ice cream: Add a spoonful of peanut butter to the blender before mixing for a nutty taste.

Strawberry banana ice cream: Add frozen strawberries to the blender before churning for a delicious taste.

Cinnamon banana ice cream: Add a teaspoon of cinnamon to the blender before mixing for a warm and comfortable taste.

After the banana ice cream is mixed to your preferred consistency, serve immediately as soft-serve or freeze for a firmer texture. You may also top it with your favorite toppings, such as chopped almonds, shredded coconut, or fresh fruit.

As a youngster, Lucy adored visiting the ice cream truck in her neighborhood during the summer. Nevertheless, when she got older and began to control her nutrition, she discovered that ice cream wasn't the healthiest choice. One day, she came across a banana ice cream recipe and decided to try it. She was delighted at how easy and tasty it was, and she enjoyed that it was a healthy alternative to typical ice cream. Today, anytime she's seeking something sweet and delicious, she makes herself a scoop of banana ice cream and reminisces about her childhood while enjoying her guilt-free pleasure.

7.3 Dark Chocolate Recipes

Dark chocolate is a tasty and healthful ingredient that can be utilized in several dessert dishes. Here are a few dishes that demonstrate the richness and depth of dark chocolate flavor:

Dark Chocolate Truffles: These bite-sized chocolates are simple to create and excellent for gratifying your sweet taste. Melt dark chocolate in a double boiler, add a dash of heavy cream, and let the mixture cool. After it has firmed, shape the chocolate into little balls and sprinkle them with cocoa powder or chopped almonds.

Dark Chocolate Brownies: Brownies are usually a crowd-pleaser, and the addition of dark chocolate elevates them to the next level. Mix melted dark chocolate, butter, sugar, and eggs, then whisk in flour and cocoa powder. Bake in a greased baking dish until set and served warm.

Dark Chocolate Bark: This simple recipe includes melting dark chocolate and spreading it on parchment paper. Sprinkle with toppings like chopped nuts, dried fruit, or sea salt, and let the chocolate firm in the refrigerator. Split the bark into bite-sized pieces and enjoy.

Dark Chocolate Mousse: For a sumptuous dessert, beat heavy cream and sugar until firm peaks form, then stir in melted dark chocolate. Chill the mixture until it sets, then serve topped with fresh berries or whipped cream.

Dark Chocolate Covered Strawberries: Dip fresh strawberries into melted dark chocolate and let them cool on wax paper. After the chocolate has solidified, these exquisite sweets are ready to enjoy.

These dark chocolate dishes are excellent for special occasions or simply as a treat to indulge in. Dark chocolate is also strong in antioxidants and may give some health advantages in moderation.

Dark chocolate truffles are a delicious and exquisite delicacy that can be produced with only a few basic ingredients. Here's a recipe that generates around 20 truffles:

Ingredients:

- 8 ounces of dark chocolate (70% or higher)
- 1/2 cup of heavy cream
- One tablespoon of unsalted butter
- Cacao powder, chopped almonds, or coconut flakes for rolling (optional) (optional)

Instructions:

1. Break the dark chocolate into tiny pieces and put them in a heatproof basin.

2. In a small saucepan, boil the heavy cream and butter over low heat until the butter is melted and the cream is just beginning to simmer.

3. Pour the hot cream mixture over the chocolate and set it for 1-2 minutes.

4. Use a spatula to whisk the mixture until the chocolate is totally melted and smooth.

5. Cover the bowl with plastic wrap and refrigerate for 2-3 hours or until the mixture is hard enough to scoop.

6. Use a tiny cookie or spoon to scoop out pieces of the batter and form them into balls.

7. If preferred, roll the truffles in cocoa powder, chopped nuts, or coconut flakes.

8. Refrigerate the truffles until ready to serve.

These dark chocolate truffles are excellent for special occasions, as a present, or as a special treat for yourself. Enjoy!

7.3.2 Dark Chocolate Brownies

Dark chocolate brownies are a delectable dish that may fulfill any chocolate lover's appetite. Here's an easy recipe for dark chocolate brownies:

Ingredients:

- 1/2 cup unsalted butter
- 1 cup granulated sugar
- Two big eggs
- One teaspoon of vanilla extract
- 1/2 cup all-purpose flour
- 1/2 cup unsweetened cocoa powder
- 1/4 teaspoon baking powder
- 1/4 teaspoon salt
- 1/2 cup dark chocolate chips

Instructions:

1. Preheat the oven to 350°F (180°C).

2. In a small saucepan, melt the butter over low heat.

3. Whisk together the sugar, eggs, and vanilla extract in a mixing dish.

4. Add the melted butter to the mixing bowl and whisk until fully incorporated.

5. Whisk together the flour, cocoa powder, baking powder, and salt in a separate mixing bowl.

6. Gradually add the dry ingredients to the wet mixture and whisk until mixed.

7. Fold in the dark chocolate chips.

8. Spoon the batter into a greased 8x8-inch baking dish.

9. Bake for 20-25 minutes or until a toothpick inserted in the middle comes out clean.

10. Let the brownies set in the pan for 10 minutes before slicing and serving.

Variations:

- Add chopped nuts or dried fruit to the dough for extra texture and flavor.

- Swirl in a spoonful of peanut butter or caramel sauce before baking for a wonderful variation.

- Garnish the cooked brownies with a sprinkle of powdered sugar or a dollop of vanilla ice cream for an extra decadent treat.

7.3.3 Dark Chocolate Mousse

Dark chocolate mousse is a delectable treat that is rich and creamy but surprisingly simple to create. Here's a recipe to create dark chocolate mousse:

Ingredients:

- 8 ounces dark chocolate, chopped
- 1/2 cup thick cream
- Two egg yolks
- 1/4 cup granulated sugar
- 1/4 cup water
- 1 tsp vanilla extract
- 1 1/2 cups whipped cream

Possible toppings: fresh berries, chopped almonds, whipped cream

Instructions:

- Melt the chocolate in a double boiler or the microwave, stirring until smooth.

- Mix the sugar and water in a small saucepan and boil over medium heat, stirring until the sugar dissolves. After dissolved, stop stirring and bring the mixture to a boil. Let it simmer for 2-3 minutes or until it gets syrupy.

- In a separate dish, whisk the egg yolks until they turn pale and thick.

- Carefully pour the boiling syrup into the egg yolks, stirring continually to prevent frying the eggs.

- Add the vanilla extract to the egg mixture and whisk until incorporated.

- Pour the egg mixture over the melted chocolate and whisk until mixed.

- In another dish, beat the heavy cream until it forms firm peaks.

- Carefully incorporate the whipped cream into the chocolate mixture until well-mixed.

- Pour the mousse into individual serving plates and refrigerate in the refrigerator for at least an hour or until set.

- After set, decorate with toppings of your choice, such as fresh berries or chopped almonds.

Enjoy your delicious and creamy dark chocolate mousse!

7.3.4 Dark Chocolate Coated Strawberries:

Dark chocolate-wrapped strawberries are a wonderful and luxurious treat that is surprisingly simple to create. Here's a recipe:

Ingredients:

- 1 pound. fresh strawberries, cleaned and dried

- Eight oz. dark chocolate chips or chopped dark chocolate

- 1 tbsp. Coconut oil (optional) (optional)

Instructions:

- Line a baking sheet with parchment paper.

- Put over a saucepan of boiling water in a double boiler or heatproof dish, and melt the dark chocolate chips or chopped chocolate until smooth. If desired, pour one tablespoon of coconut oil to produce a smoother, shinier chocolate coating.

- After the chocolate is melted, could you remove it from the fire?

- Take each strawberry by the stem and dip it into the melted chocolate, swirling to cover it evenly.

- Carefully shake off any excess chocolate, then lay the strawberry on the prepared baking sheet.

- Continue with the remaining strawberries, and put the baking sheet in the refrigerator to enable the chocolate to solidify.

- After the chocolate has solidified, the strawberries are ready to serve.

Variations:

- Pour melted white chocolate over the dark chocolate-covered strawberries for an elegant and delectable touch.

- Crushed nuts or sprinkles may be added to the chocolate coating for extra texture and taste.

- Add food coloring to tint the white chocolate pink or red for Valentine's Day or other special occasions for a fun and festive touch.

Dark chocolate-wrapped strawberries are a classic and romantic delicacy commonly linked with Valentine's Day or other special events. They make a nice and decadent present for a loved one or maybe savored as a sumptuous treat any time of year. Creating them at home is easy and entertaining to wow visitors or show someone you care.

8.0 Food Planning and Prep Ideas for PCOS

8.1 Batch Cooking and Freezing Suggestions

Batch cooking and freezing are fantastic strategies to save time and money while ensuring you have healthful meals readily accessible. Here are some guidelines for good batch cooking and freezing:

Plan ahead: Pick recipes that freeze well and develop a shopping list to ensure you have all the required supplies.

Invest in quality containers: Choose freezer-safe, airtight, and stackable containers to optimize space in your freezer.

Label everything: Label your containers with the name of the food, the date it was produced, and any reheating instructions.

Freeze in portions: Freeze meals in individual portions or family-sized quantities for simple thawing and reheating.

Cool before freezing: Let your food cool to room temperature before freezing to avoid condensation and freezer burn.

Utilize freezer-friendly ingredients: Certain items, such as dairy-based sauces or crops with high water content, don't freeze well. Adhere to foods like grains, beans, meats, and stews that freeze well.

Maintain a freezer inventory: Keep track of what you have in the freezer to prevent overstocking or losing track of what has to be consumed.

Here are some examples of dishes that freeze well:

Soups and stews: Vegetable soup, chili, lentil soup, meat stew

Casseroles: Lasagna, baked ziti, shepherd's pie Proteins: Cooked chicken, ground beef, meatballs

Grains and pasta: Quinoa, rice, pasta recipes like spaghetti and meatballs or baked mac and cheese

Baked goods: Muffins, bread, cookies

Following these recommendations and picking the perfect dishes to freeze, bulk cooking and freezing may be game-changers for hectic weeknights.

8.2 How to Eat Out and Adhere to Your PCOS Diet

Polycystic ovarian syndrome (PCOS) is a common hormonal disease in women that may lead to many health difficulties, including weight gain, insulin resistance, and reproductive problems. Maintaining a healthy diet is an essential part of managing PCOS symptoms. However, eating out can be challenging, as finding healthy options that fit into a PCOS-friendly diet can be difficult. Here are some tips for eating out and sticking to your PCOS diet:

Research the restaurant: Before heading out, research the restaurant you plan to visit. Check out the menu online and look for options that fit into your PCOS diet, such as grilled chicken or fish with vegetables, salads, and soups.

Make modifications:
1. Feel free to make modifications to your meal.
2. Ask for dressings.
3. Put sauces on the side, swap vegetables for rice or pasta, and ask for grilled or baked alternatives instead of fried.

Beware of hidden sugars: Many restaurant entrees, particularly savory ones, might include hidden sugars. Be wary of sugary sauces, dressings, and marinades. Select foods with basic ingredients and avoid processed or pre-packaged meals.

Control portions: Restaurant servings are typically greater than what we require. Try splitting an entrée with a buddy, ask for a to-go box, and store half of your meal for later.

Be wary of alcohol: Alcohol may be heavy in calories and sugar and interfere with insulin sensitivity. Go for low-sugar choices like wine or spirits blended with soda water, and restrict yourself to one drink.

Don't be too harsh on yourself: Dining out doesn't have to be flawless. If you indulge in a less-than-healthy lunch, don't beat yourself up. Go back on track with your PCOS diet the following day and concentrate on progress rather than perfection.

Following these recommendations, you may enjoy dining out while maintaining your PCOS-friendly diet.

9.0 Resources and Help for PCOS

9.1 PCOS-Friendly Food and Supplement Recommendations

Supplement advice may be useful for persons with particular health issues, such as PCOS, to support their general health and well-being. It's crucial to remember that supplements should not replace a balanced diet and regular exercise but may complement these lifestyle improvements.

For PCOS, some often prescribed nutrients include:

Inositol: Inositol is a form of carbohydrate that may help improve insulin resistance and hormone balance in women with PCOS. It may also aid with weight reduction and fertility. The two most prevalent types of inositol utilized for PCOS are Myo-inositol and D-chiro inositol.

Omega-3 fatty acids: Omega-3 fatty acids are anti-inflammatory and may help decrease inflammation in the body, which can be good for women with PCOS who have inflammation-related symptoms such as acne and irregular periods.

Vitamin D: Vitamin D has a role in insulin sensitivity and hormone balance, and many women with PCOS lack this mineral. Supplementation may help symptoms such as menstrual irregularity and hirsutism (excess hair growth) (excess hair growth).

N-acetyl cysteine (NAC): NAC is an antioxidant that may help improve insulin sensitivity, decrease inflammation, and regulate menstrual cycles in women with PCOS.

Chromium: Chromium is a mineral that might help improve insulin sensitivity and glucose metabolism, thereby alleviating symptoms of PCOS such as acne, weight gain, and irregular periods.

It's crucial to check with a healthcare practitioner before beginning any new supplement program since certain supplements might interfere with prescriptions or have possible negative effects.

It's also crucial to buy high-quality supplements from reliable vendors.

Here are some extra readings and websites that might give further knowledge and help for specific dietary needs:

Academy of Nutrition and Dietetics: This organization offers consumers and healthcare professionals evidence-based nutrition information and tools.

American Diabetes Association: The ADA offers services and assistance for persons with diabetes and their families.

The Whole30 Program: This program is a 30-day dietary reset meant to help people discover and remove items that may harm their health adversely.

The Low FODMAP Diet: This diet is meant to assist persons with digestive problems, including irritable bowel syndrome (IBS), in lowering their consumption of fermentable carbohydrates.

National Celiac Association: This group offers information and support for those with celiac disease and gluten sensitivity.

Plant-Based Nutrition: This website offers information and resources for anyone interested in a plant-based diet.

Vegetarian Resource Group: This group offers information and assistance for anyone interested in a vegetarian or vegan lifestyle.

The Ketogenic Diet: This high-fat, low-carbohydrate diet has been demonstrated to offer advantages for weight reduction and some medical issues.

The Mediterranean Diet: This diet is based on the typical eating habits of nations surrounding the Mediterranean Sea and has been connected with several health advantages.

MyFitnessPal: This software and website enable users to log their food consumption and assess their progress towards their health objectives.

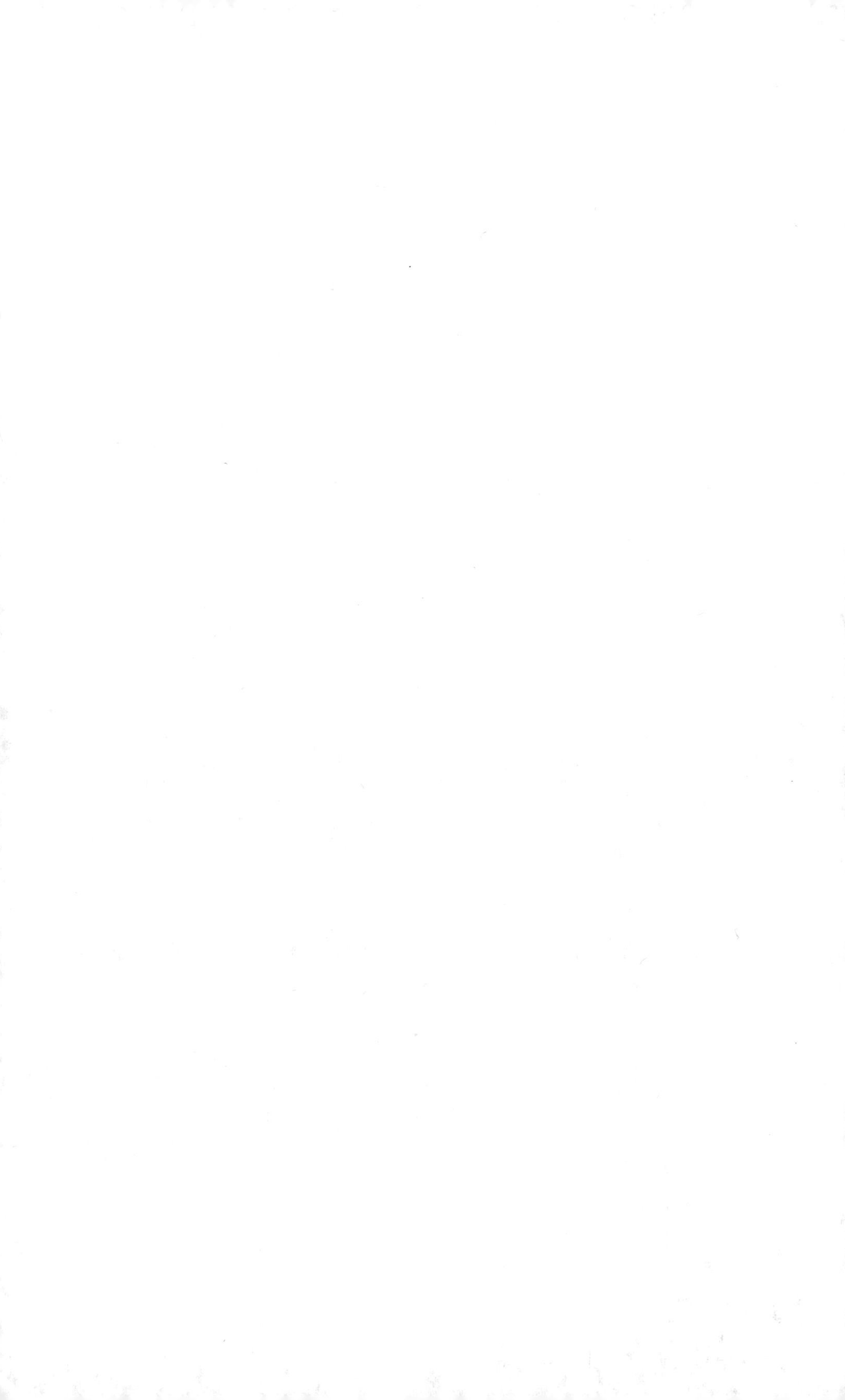